Pregnancy and Bipolar Disorder

Estevan Cavalcanti

Abstract

Bipolar disorder (BD) affects a significant proportion of women. Although a considerable amount of information is available to the public regarding the general treatment of BD, and although there has been a considerable amount of recent research about the treatment of BD during pregnancy that is aimed at healthcare providers, little information geared toward women with BD is available on the comprehensive and holistic management of BD during pregnancy. The purpose of this study was to learn about women with BD's concerns and experiences related to pregnancy issues. Thirty-eight participants, including 20 women who reported being diagnosed with BD-I, and 18 women who reported being diagnosed with BD-II, participated in an open-ended online questionnaire ($n = 31$) or telephone survey ($n = 7$) which inquired about their concerns, fears, desired information, advice, and experiences related to BD and pregnancy. Qualitative thematic analysis identified six key findings: (a) women of childbearing years diagnosed with BD are profoundly concerned about pregnancy issues; (b) women with BD are afraid of harming their unborn children and babies; (c) women with BD are eager to educate themselves about pregnancy issues, and they are dissatisfied with the information they are finding; (d) women with BD want their healthcare providers to inform them of the risks associated with various treatment options during pregnancy, as well as pregnancy and mood issues; (e) women with BD recommend and desire psychotherapy during pregnancy, and they want to know how to include their partners in therapy; and (f) women with BD are concerned about their relationships with their healthcare providers.

Key words: Bipolar disorder, pregnancy, women, qualitative research

Table of Contents

Chapter I

Introduction

All women must face the inevitable reality that becoming a mother involves setting aside one's own needs for those of one's child. When a woman has bipolar disorder (BD), an illness experienced by an estimated 1 in every 100 women, the repercussions of failing to address her needs can potentially include relationship conflicts, worse mood symptoms, suicide, and infanticide (Yonkers et al., 2004). Women with BD also often worry that they will not be good enough parents and that they will pass their disorder on to their children (Blegen, Hummelvoll, & Severinsson, 2010). Concerns about pregnancy among women with BD are likely to be common and are likely to begin long before they decide whether or not to become pregnant.

Although a considerable amount of information is available to the public regarding the general treatment of BD, little information is available on the comprehensive and holistic management of BD during pregnancy. The most common advice given to women considering becoming pregnant is that they should consult with a psychiatrist. This lack of available information is a disservice to women with BD. Such information is crucial for a woman and her partner to realistically consider risks and benefits, identify warning signs of mood episodes, and manage the pregnancy and postpartum period.

Although there is a dearth of information available to the general public, there has been a good deal of research and clinical guidelines aimed at healthcare providers that address this issue, such as, "What's the Best Strategy for Bipolar Disorder During Pregnancy?" (Minick & Atlas, 200) and "Management of Bipolar Disorder During

Pregnancy and the Postpartum Period" (Yonkers et al., 2004). These publications focus almost universally on medication management of BD and risks and benefits of medication management to the mother and fetus. These publications have mostly been produced by physicians for physicians rather than for nonphysician mental health providers. The field of clinical psychology has an enormous potential contribution to make to this literature relevant to considerations of planning and managing a pregnancy with BD. It can provide unique perspectives and behavioral strategies, which can create a more complete, usable, and useful body of knowledge. There is a need to translate mental health interventions and existing research into a vehicle that is accessible to nonmedical professionals and nonprofessionals. This study aims to learn about the kind of information, services and support that women with BD need related to pregnancy.

The second chapter of this dissertation reviews relevant research and clinical thought that provides the foundation for a psychology-informed management of BD in pregnancy. This will begin with discussion of research on the major pregnancy issues that women with BD face across prenatal, pregnancy, and postpartum periods. This includes the incidence of new mood episodes and teratogenic effects of various drugs used to treat BD during the planning, pregnancy, and postpartum stages of pregnancy. A discussion of the existing literature on interventions used to prevent mood episodes and how they can be applied to pregnant women with BD will follow.

The third chapter of this dissertation, the Methods, describes the methodology for a survey of women with BD to learn about their perspectives on pregnancy issues. The fourth and fifth chapters of this dissertation provide the results of this study as well as a discussion of the findings, respectively. It is hoped that this study will bring greater attention to the issues related to having BD and becoming pregnant or considering

becoming pregnant, and that this will help women with BD to more thoughtfully make

decisions related to pregnancy.

Chapter II

Literature Review

Overview of BD and the Stages of Pregnancy

Epidemiology. BD affects an estimated 0.5%-1.5% of individuals in the United States (Yonkers, et. al, 2004). Men and women are equally likely to have this illness, although women are more likely to have the rapid-cycling form (more than 4 episodes per year) and are also more likely to experience depressive symptoms and mixed states (Stowe & Newport, 2007). Women are typically diagnosed with BD during their teens and early 20s, which place them at risk for mood episodes during their reproductive years. Given that 82% of women in the United States have children by the age of 44, it is clear that issues of conception, pregnancy, and postpartum periods are of great relevance to the topic of BD among women (Taylor et al., 2010). There is a nearly sevenfold higher risk of admission for a first episode of BD and a nearly twofold higher risk for a recurrent episode in postpartum women compared to nonpregnant and nonpostpartum women with BD (Yonkers, et. al, 2004). Many of the medications used to treat BD pose known or unknown risks to the fetus and infant if they are used during pregnancy or breastfeeding. However, discontinuation of medication poses considerable risk as well. For example, women with BD who discontinue lithium therapy during the postpartum period are three times more likely to have a mood episode at this time than their nonpregnant counterparts (Stowe & Newport, 2007).

Impact of mood episodes during the stages of pregnancy. Eighty percent of mood episodes experienced by women with BD during pregnancy or the postpartum period are of the depressive or mixed variety (Viguera, 2007). Only 20% are manic or hypomanic episodes in these stages of pregnancy. This indicates that any intervention must take into account the potential of a woman with BD experiencing both depressed and manic states. Studies indicate that even modest maternal depression or stress can adversely affect infant wellbeing (Stowe & Newport, 2007). Impaired judgment and impulsivity are symptoms of untreated mania that often result in poor self-care, which is dangerous to both mother and child (Freeman, 2007). Untreated mania and depression increase the likelihood of risky behavior and substance use, which can result in negative consequences for both the mother and fetus (Curtis, 2005). Risky behaviors may include suicide and impulsive decisions to terminate pregnancy. The overall suicide rate among those with BD is estimated at 15%; the rate of suicide among those with untreated BD is 25 times higher than that of the general population (Rihmer, 2009). Suicides occur most often during severe depressive episodes. Women experiencing severe mood episodes during pregnancy may need to be hospitalized. Hospitalization could result in the fetus's exposure to multiple psychotropic medications at relatively high doses, which increases the risk of harmful medication effects (Viguera, Cohen, Baldessarini, & Nonacs, 2002). Deterioration in mental state can also affect a woman's ability to bond with, and parent, her child (Kulkarni et al., 2008). Infanticide is a well-documented risk of postpartum psychosis (Kim, Choi, & Ha, 2008). In addition, mood episodes put a great deal of stress on the mother with BD, her partner, and their family.

Mental health treatment goals for BD relative to stage of pregnancy.

Mental health treatment goals common to all stages of pregnancy. This dissertation separately considered three stages of pregnancy: the preconception or planning stage, the prenatal or pregnancy stage, and the postpartum or post-delivery stage. However, a number of treatment goals are common to all stages. From the practitioner's perspective, these goals include the need to provide education to the woman with BD and her partner, engaging the woman, her loved ones, and practitioners to monitor for new mood symptoms, and reducing mood episodes to zero (Barnes & Mitchell, 2005; Frieder, Dunlop, Culpepper, & Bernstein, 2008). From the perspective of the woman with BD, goals throughout the preconception, pregnancy, and the postpartum periods include educating herself as much as possible regarding the way BD may affect pregnancy, avoiding stress, getting adequate sleep, monitoring her mood and symptoms, maintaining good physical and mental health, and asking for help when it is needed (Ward & Wisner, 2007; Yonkers, et al., 2004). It is also recommended that she establish a strong and stable therapeutic alliance with physicians and relevant practitioners (such as the family practitioner, the obstetrician-gynecologist, the psychiatrist, and the psychologist). Kristin Finn, author of *Bipolar and Pregnant*, (2007) stated the following:

> Your relationships with your OB-GYN and psychiatrist are a crucial part of your pregnancy. As a [woman with BD], you have a unique situation, and I can't stress enough how important it is for you to feel comfortable and confident with your doctors. Working with professionals who are empathetic is wonderful. Keep looking until you find the right match for you. (p. 127)

Of course, the usual recommendations for all pregnant women and those attempting to become pregnant also apply. The Centers for Disease Control and Prevention recommend women avoid alcohol, nicotine, and other substances, take prenatal vitamins, maintain a healthy diet, exercise, and avoid obesity (2010).

Mental health treatment goals specific to the preconception period. The overall treatment goals for women with BD during this period are to avoid unplanned pregnancies, ensure that health professionals are aware of and involved with planning the pregnancy, and to reduce the fetus's exposure to teratogenic medications that are often used as preventative treatments for BD (Frieder et al., 2008).

The importance of planned pregnancies among women with BD. Christina Marie Bailey (2008), author of an autobiographical book describing her experience of having an unplanned pregnancy as a woman with BD, stated the following:

> When I first faced the reality that I would be on psychiatric medication for the rest of my life, I struggled with the fact that pregnancy would be, at the very least, difficult. I was twenty-one years old. Although there was always a small part of me that longed to have a child of my own, I had come to accept that I would never go through pregnancy . . . or so I thought . . . . I began to feel that I could not, that I was in fact, incapable of, getting pregnant. I guess that comes from past experience and that familiar feeling of invincibility that goes hand in hand with my disorder. (p. 72)

Planning their pregnancies is one of the most important things women with BD can do to increase their odds of having positive pregnancy outcomes (Curtis, 2005; Newport et al., 2008). However, only about half of all pregnancies among all women in the United States are planned (Finer & Henshaw, 2006). Manic or hypomanic episodes often include sexual activity of a highly risky nature that gives rise to a significant risk of unplanned pregnancy (Frieder et al., 2008). Thus, many doctors recommend that women with BD use contraception until they are truly ready to conceive (Curtis, 2005).

Women with BD should be aware that some medications used to treat BD, in particular antiepileptic medications, interact with oral contraceptives. The antiepileptic agents carbamazepine (Tegretol®), oxcarbazepine (Trileptal®), and topiramate (Topamax®) all increase the clearance rate of oral contraceptives, thereby increasing the likelihood of pregnancy (Curtis, 2005). Women with BD using these drugs are recommended to use a higher oral contraceptive dose, a second contraceptive method, or a different contraceptive method altogether. Some oral contraceptives increase the clearance rate of drugs, such as lamotrigine, used to treat BD (Ward & Wisner, 2007). Women with BD who are considering using oral contraceptives should discuss this issue with their doctors before they begin. Their doctors may opt to increase their bipolar medication dosage.

The first trimester is the time when the fetus is at greatest risk of being negatively affected by teratogenic medications, which includes those that are used to treat BD (Viguera, 2007). Many women do not find out they are pregnant until well into this critical period, and at that point their fetuses will have already been exposed. Thus, the issue of pregnancy and medication risk to their fetus should be discussed with all women with BD of childbearing potential, regardless of their future reproductive plans. Treatment planning should take place before the woman is pregnant, while she is free of mood symptoms, which could cloud her judgment (Barnes & Mitchell, 2005).

The decision to continue or stop taking medication. Deciding to switch or stop medication therapy for BD during pregnancy causes many women to feel scared (Viguera, Cohen, Baldessarini et al., 2002). They may worry that they will go crazy, ruin their relationship with their partner, or never feel as healthy again, even if medication is resumed. Choosing to stay on medication during pregnancy also seems like it would cause a lot of fear and guilt. Women may worry that they will damage their unborn children. They may feel selfish and guilty for not sacrificing their sanity; they may feel ashamed that they are not strong enough to get through pregnancy without medication.

This can reactivate feelings of grief over the "lost healthy self" that so many people with BD experience. Kristin Finn, in her personal memoir, opted to forego medication during pregnancy. She recalled that, "As I prepared to discontinue lithium to become pregnant, I was terrified. Can you imagine going off a medication that has sustained your sanity? I hadn't experienced the intense, ongoing symptoms of mania and depression in more than ten years" (Finn, 2007, p. 31). Pressure from partners and family members to avoid medication during pregnancy may make women with BD feel as though they alone and judged by others. Psychotherapy may be helpful for women with BD who are planning a pregnancy, because it can help them better understand and manage the complex feelings that are likely to emerge concerning medication use or disuse.

Clinical guidelines strongly recommend that women avoid becoming pregnant until their BD is in remission (Barnes & Mitchell, 2005; Frieder, et al., 2008). There is evidence that women who have been in remission longer are less likely to have a new mood episode during pregnancy (Newport et al., 2008; Viguera et al., 2007). Physicians should take into account several factors when developing an individualized plan for the treatment of women with BD who are planning a pregnancy: each individual woman's prior response to medication, length of time she is mood episode-free while taking and not taking medication, time to relapse after medication discontinuation, and time to recover with reintroduction of medication (Yonkers et al., 2004). Women with BD should be aware of these factors and work with their doctors to make an informed decision about whether or not to conceive.

According to Viguera (2005), women should probably not discontinue medication during their pregnancies if they have had a history of multiple episodes (more than 3 or 4) and if they have required hospitalization or have become suicidal when they were symptomatic. She indicates that women should not discontinue their medication if they do not get well between episodes, if they become very ill when they have an episode, or if they immediately enter a psychotic manic state or become severely depressed. Practitioners of women with severe BD may elect to encourage them to continue taking medication while they attempt to conceive. In order to avoid teratogenic risks to the fetus, practitioners may opt to switch women with BD to older antipsychotic medications or to risperidone, which appear to be safer for the fetus (Yonkers et al., 2004). Unfortunately, these medications increase prolactin levels, thereby decreasing menstrual cyclicity, which has a negative impact on fertility. Women who are in remission from BD and have less severe illness histories may be able to discontinue taking a mood stabilizer before attempting to conceive; however, according to Yonkers and colleagues, physicians should ensure that their medication dosage is tapered slowly because discontinuation of maintenance medication is associated with high rates of relapse, especially if discontinuation occurs abruptly (Yonkers et. al, 2004).

Genetic counseling. BD is believed to be partially heritable, and genetic counseling may benefit women who want to learn more about the likelihood of conceiving offspring with BD or related emotional conditions (Minick & Atlas, 2007). Paterson, Parker, Fletcher and Graham (2013) of the Sydney, Australia Black Dog Institute Depression Clinic conducted a study to compare views about pregnancy among women diagnosed with depression with those diagnosed with BD. Four hundred and two women participated by completing an eight-statement questionnaire with a 5-point rating scale. They found that women with BD were more concerned than women with unipolar depression regarding the way pregnancy would affect their mood, as well as the risk of passing their condition on to their children.

The information a genetic counselor provides may help some women decide whether or not to have children biologically. Trippitelli et al. (1998) conducted a survey of 90 people with BD and their unaffected spouses on genetic counseling. Results indicated that among those with BD and their spouses who were surveyed, if such tests were available, approximately 44% would probably or definitely test a fetus for BD, whereas 40% reported they would not. About 16% reported that they were unsure whether they would have a fetus tested or not. When participants were asked if they would abort a fetus that carried a gene for BD, 55% of those with BD and 65% of their spouses said that they would definitely not abort a fetus for this reason.

The risk for BD among first-degree relatives of a patient with BD has been estimated to range from 1.5%-10.2%, and the risk is believed to be elevated for the offspring of a parent with early-onset BD (onset at 17 years or younger; Curtis, 2005). An expert on the treatment of BD during pregnancy, Adele Viguera, M.D., stated that circumstances in which it would be appropriate for a clinician to advise against pregnancy are "quite rare" (Viguera, 2005). However, she reported that in one study, 45% of women diagnosed with BD who underwent genetic counseling were advised not to conceive (Viguera, 2005). She noted that women with BD should be warned that the stigma associated with their disease could color genetic counselors' opinions about their reproductive plans.

Mental health treatment goals specific to the prenatal period. Many women with BD have posted their experiences and concerns regarding pregnancy on message boards and web logs via the Internet. For example, on a Facebook support group for pregnant women and mothers with BD, members often write about their difficult mood symptoms, frustration with their healthcare providers, and request and give each other advice on how to change their medication regimens ("Bipolar, Depressed, and Pregnant or a Mother," 2013). Many women report having been worried that they might suffer from new mood disorders while pregnant, but that they eventually make it through the pregnancy with normal mood or with minimal shifts in mood (Hoos, 2009; Rachael, 2007). Michelle Roberts of *Bp Magazine* (2013) published a story about a woman with BD who had a very difficult pregnancy:

> With input from her doctor, Candace eased off her antipsychotic medication, but stayed on lithium "with the hope that I would stay well and the baby wouldn't be harmed." Then something unexpected happened. During her first trimester, she experienced excessive vomiting and couldn't keep down her lithium. While she was hospitalized for her physical symptoms, she had a full-blown manic episode. "I was completely delusional," she says. "I was screaming out at times. A psychiatric resident walked into my room and I attacked him. Once they got the vomiting stabilized, I was transferred to the psychiatric unit" (para. 8).

Candace's presentation was unusual, as most mood episodes that occur in women with BD during pregnancy are of the depressive type (Viguera, 2007).

Important treatment goals for all pregnant women, including all women with BD, include having an obstetrician involved with the pregnancy and adhering to a schedule of prenatal care visits with them (Viguera, 2004). Viguera recommends that first-time mothers should also attend childbirth preparation classes. Specific treatment goals for women with BD during this period are to minimize teratogenic risks to the fetus and to manage the bipolar illness. Viguera et al. (2011) analyzed data from over 2000 women diagnosed with BD-I, BD-II, or recurrent major depressive disorder and found that 23% of women diagnosed with BD experienced a mood episode during pregnancy. In addition, younger age at illness onset was the factor most highly correlated with experiencing a mood episode during pregnancy. Not being married was also associated with mood episodes experienced during pregnancy. In a separate study of new mood episodes that occurred among pregnant women with BD, 47.2%, 31.9%, and 18.8% occurred during the first, second, and third trimester, respectively (Viguera, 2007). In keeping with the findings of the study cited above, the periods of highest risk for mood episode during pregnancy are usually during the first trimester (Yonkers, et. al, 2004). Due to risk of teratogenic effects of medication, many physicians may work with women to help them discontinue medication use either while they are trying to become pregnant or when they learn they are pregnant. Women with BD who discontinue using their medication before pregnancy or during the first trimester and do not experience mood symptoms may be encouraged not to restart medication until later in the pregnancy, should they notice early signs of relapse (Ward & Wisner, 2007). The physicians of women with histories of self-harm, impaired insight, a long recovery time, or evidence that their support system cannot deal with another mood episode may choose to encourage them to re-start medication regardless of their symptoms after the first trimester ends, in order to increase the odds that they do not relapse (Yonkers et al., 2004).

Should the treating professional feel that it is warranted that a woman continue to take medication during the first trimester, one article recommended that it is best that the woman use only one medication at the lowest therapeutic dosage (Burt & Rasgon, 2004). The authors noted that medication that poses the least teratogenic risk should be prescribed. Older medications are preferred because more data is available on their safety compared to newer drugs (Viguera, Cohen, Baldessarini et al., 2002). The treating practitioner may choose to disregard this advice if his or her patient has a hard-to-treat case of BD, and the effectiveness of a certain medication they have been taking justifies fetal exposure to the drug for that particular patient (Viguera, Cohen, Baldessarini et al., 2002).

Hormonal changes during the prenatal period. According to the American Pregnancy Association's (2013) website:

> Significant changes in your hormone levels can affect your level of neurotransmitters, which are brain chemicals that regulate mood. Mood swings are mostly experienced during the first trimester between 6 to 10 weeks and then again in the third trimester as your body prepares for birth (para. 3).

They add that women with BD should be educated about the way their changing pregnancy hormone levels may affect their mood.

Treatment goals specific to the postpartum period. Of all the life stages of a woman with BD, the postpartum period is the riskiest time for the exacerbation of BD (Curtis, 2005). Hunt and Silverstone (1995) reported that women with BD have a 25-40% chance of developing a postpartum mood episode (manic or depressive). A retrospective analysis of 2,134 women with BD from the nationwide Swedish Medical Birth and Hospital Discharge register revealed that 5.15% of women hospitalized for an episode of BD at any point before pregnancy and not prenatally had a recurrent episode during the postpartum period that required hospitalization, whereas 41.26% of those hospitalized for a bipolar episode during the prenatal period also had a postpartum recurrence that required hospitalization (Harlow et al., 2007). In their analysis of over 2000 women with unipolar or bipolar disorders, Viguera et al. (2011) found that women diagnosed with BD had a 52% chance of experiencing a postpartum mood episode. Therefore, she notes, it is very important that the mother, her partner, family, and physicians watch for new mood symptoms during this time.

Postpartum psychosis. Postpartum psychosis is defined as a postpartum manic episode, often presenting with delirium or psychotic features. Symptoms may include hallucinations, delusions, severe depression, thoughts of harming or killing oneself or one's baby, unwillingness to eat or sleep, and frantic energy (Silberner, 2002). Shelley Ash, a woman without previous history of psychiatric illness, described her experience of postpartum psychosis to a National Public Radio (NPR) reporter:

> "I knew right away something was wrong," says Ash. She sensed she was watching the delivery from above. She was terrified. Hospital nurses told her the feeling would pass. It didn't, even after she and her baby went home . . . Ash says she was pacing all the time, and caught in a horrible depression. She was constantly crying, couldn't sleep and couldn't eat . . . Ash knew she was getting worse. The midwife in her obstetrician's office told her to call a psychiatrist. . . . "I was terrified," says Ash. She was having delusions and was afraid that if she told anyone about what she was thinking or seeing in her mind, they would take her son away . . . She remembers watching David Letterman drop watermelons from high places on his television show. "But that turned into my son," she says. "I kept imagining how it would be to drop him out of his bedroom window and he would go splat on the pavement below and shatter into a million pieces." The image was too much for her. Ash went to her bathroom cabinet and took an overdose of painkillers she had been prescribed for a previous back injury. Her husband came home from a run to find her on the floor in the front hall, babbling, and he rushed her to the hospital. (Silberner, 2002, para. 3)

Among women with BD, an estimated 20-30% will experience this affliction (Viguera, 2005). In contrast, for women without BD, postpartum psychosis is rare; it occurs in only 1 in 1000 women. A suicide rate of approximately 4% and an infanticide rate of approximately 4% are associated with postpartum psychosis; thus, this condition is considered a medical emergency (Pfuhlmann, Stoeber, & Beckmann, 2002; Viguera, 2005; Yonkers et al., 2004). Studies suggest that women who have experienced one postpartum psychotic episode have a 50-90% higher risk of having a subsequent episode during their future postpartum periods (Barnes & Mitchell, 2005). More recent pre-

pregnancy hospitalizations and larger numbers of pre-pregnancy hospitalizations have been found to increase the risk of postpartum manic episodes with psychotic features (Harlow et al., 2007). The modal day that postpartum psychosis occurs is day 1, the day of delivery, so new mothers should be watched for its symptoms very closely after giving birth.

Infanticide. In a retrospective study of 33 women with BD who had killed their children, all of the women had presented with childlike behavior and *la belle indifference* (an inappropriate lack of concern about one's symptoms) shortly before doing so (Kim et al., 2008). Stanton et al. (2000) found that women who were in a state of mania when they killed their children did not demonstrate premeditation; they had developed delusions no greater than within a day before the offense. Women who were depressed at the time of the offense reported thinking about the deaths of their children for days or weeks beforehand. The women were classified into 3 groups based on their motivation to kill: (a) acute psychosis—the mother was following commanding auditory hallucinations or persecutory delusions that her children were "monsters" or "possessed by Satan" (Kim et al., 2008, p. 1626); (b) impulsivity—unexpected death was caused by anger outbursts toward her children in the form of impulsive, violent behavior; (c) confusion—the mother was confused at the time of the offense and "in whom a comprehensible motive could not be attained" (Kim et al., p. 1626). Suffocation was the most common method of murder.

Postpartum depression. Katherine Stone (2009) is an award-winning perinatal mood and anxiety disorder advocate and the author of Postpartum Progress, the most widely-read blog in the United States on postpartum depression. On her blog, she has described postpartum depression as a period of 2 weeks or more that occurs within 12 months of giving birth, in which some of the following symptoms are experienced: feeling overwhelmed, guilty, confused, scared, irritated, angry, numb, sad, and/or hopeless; feeling disconnected from one's child; changes in sleep and/or appetite; difficulty concentrating; thoughts of harming oneself or others. Postpartum depression occurs in up to 10-20% of all mothers the year following delivery (Campbell & Cohen, 1991). Less research exists regarding the prevalence of postpartum depression among women with BD. Freeman et al. (2002) found that 20 out of 30 women with BD experienced a postpartum mood episode within one month of delivery, and most of these episodes were of a depressive nature. In another study, all eight women with more than one child who experienced postpartum depression following the birth of their first child had a recurrence upon the birth of their second child (Freeman et al., 2002). Various authors have concluded that genetics, hormonal changes, sleep deprivation, and the stress of becoming a new mother are involved in at least some cases of postpartum depression; therefore, new mothers with BD should utilize treatment interventions that focus on stress reduction and adequate sleep (Yonkers et al., 2004).

Hormonal changes during the postpartum period. In a 2012 review article, Studd and Nappi discussed issues related to *reproductive depression*, which is depressed mood related to fluctuating hormone levels associated with menstruation, pregnancy, and menopause. They noted that, "Virtually every neural pathway (serotonergic, dopaminergic, noradrenergic, cholinergic, GABAergic, etc.) responds to estrogens" (p. 42), and depression occurs in women vulnerable to hormonal fluctuations when estrogen levels are low, such as during the postpartum period (McEwens & Alves, as referenced in Studd & Nappi, 2012). The authors emphasized the importance of psychiatrists accurately assessing for reproductive depression by inquiring about matters such as premenstrual depression history and relief of depression during pregnancy, so that they can treat it with estrogen replacement therapy rather than antidepressants alone. They also noted that lower estradiol levels, which are associated with breastfeeding for a longer amount of time, are correlated with more severe depression that lasts longer. Clearly, this is a complex issue which women with BD who suffer from postpartum mood issues should be made aware of.

Overview of strategies used to treat BD during pregnancy. As mentioned above, the treatment goals common to all stages of pregnancy for women with BD include educating them about the way BD affects pregnancy and helping them maintain their physical and mental health (Ward & Wisner, 2007; Yonkers, et al., 2004). During the preconception period, women with BD should strive to avoid unplanned pregnancies and ensure that their BD is in remission before planning to conceive (Barnes & Mitchell, 2005; Curtis, 2005; Frieder et al., 2008; Newport et al., 2008). Women should work with their physicians to determine which medications, if any, they will take during pregnancy (Viguera, 2005). The main goals during the prenatal period are to minimize teratogenic risks to the fetus and to manage the BD illness (Viguera, 2007). During the postpartum period, goals for women with BD include deciding whether or not to breastfeed and avoiding experiencing new mood episodes; there is greater risk than at any other time for experiencing an episode (Hunt & Silverstone, 1995).

In order to improve the likelihood of achieving these goals, women with BD are recommended to avoid stress, get adequate amounts of sleep, keep track of their mood and symptoms, and ask for help from their partner and support network (Ward & Wisner,

2007; Yonkers, et al., 2004). The Centers for Disease Control and Prevention (CDC, 2011) recommends that all pregnant women avoid substance use, take prenatal vitamins, maintain a healthy diet and exercise regularly in order to improve pregnancy outcome. The most frequent day postpartum psychosis occurs is the day of delivery, so new mothers should enlist the help of their partners and those close to them to help recognize early warning signs of this condition and report them to their physicians (Viguera, 2005). Various authors have concluded that sleep deprivation and the stress of becoming a new mother are likely involved in at least some cases of postpartum depression; therefore, new mothers with BD should utilize treatment interventions that focus on stress reduction and adequate sleep (Yonkers et al., 2004).

Psychotropic drugs are commonly used to prevent pregnant women with BD from experiencing new mood episodes. There is a growing body of evidence outlining recommendations regarding medication dosages and which agents are less harmful to the developing infant. The next section will discuss this topic in detail. Much less research has been conducted regarding behavioral and psychotherapeutic interventions for the management of BD during pregnancy provided either in tandem with medication or without medication. This is not surprising, given the risks associated with this population and the difficulty in designing studies that would not violate the ethical standards on research with human subjects. Currently, general recommendations are limited to lifestyle changes such as reducing stress, getting adequate amounts of sleep, and getting regular exercise. The third section of this chapter will provide more details on this subject, as well as information on prospective psychotherapeutic and complementary medicine interventions that have not been tested on pregnant women with BD but could potentially prove helpful.

Medication

General considerations. A 2001 survey suggested that regardless of their education, socioeconomic status, or the characteristics of the physicians who treat them, women with BD are often poorly informed about the risks that psychotropic drug exposure poses to the fetus, as well as the high rates of relapse during pregnancy and the postpartum period when psychotropic drug treatment is discontinued (Viguera, Cohen, Bouffard, et al., 2002). Psychotropic medication passes through the placenta (Viguera, Cohen, Bouffard, et al., 2002). Seeman (2004) stated that unborn babies are potentially more susceptible to drug effects because their liver enzymes are less available to metabolically inactivate medication, and because their nervous systems are not fully developed. The risk of fetal malformation as a result of a woman with BD's medication use depends on the drug's properties and the time period of the fetus's exposure (Yonkers et al., 2004). According to Yonkers et al. (2004), "Exposure up to 32 days after conception can affect neural tube development and closure; exposure 21-56 days after conception may affect heart formation; and exposure during days 42-63 may influence development of the lip and palate" (p. 609). Craniofacial anomalies and neurobehavioral teratogenicity can also result from exposure after the first trimester.

Side effects and efficacy of medications used to treat and prevent BD vary from person to person (Ward & Wisner, 2007). Thus, a number of different medications have been developed and are prescribed for the prevention and treatment of BD mood episodes. Some medications are used in combination with others. The most commonly prescribed drugs for the treatment and prophylaxis of BD are lithium, anticonvulsants, and antipsychotics. Each medication has a different safety profile regarding its use during pregnancy and lactation.

Specific medications and teratogenicity.

Lithium. Congenital malformations are the main risk associated with fetal exposure to lithium. The most common malformation associated with lithium exposure is a heart defect called Ebstein's anomaly, which is associated with 100% mortality in its most severe form. It occurs at a rate of 1 in 20,000 infants in the general population compared to 1-2 in 1,000 infants exposed to lithium in utero (Yonkers, et al., 2004). This risk is quite low overall, and many women at high risk for BD relapse are counseled to continue taking the medication during the 2nd and 3rd trimesters and sometimes the first as well (Viguera, 2005). *Floppy baby syndrome*, characterized by blue skin coloring and less muscle tone and tension than usual is the most common toxicity effect in babies exposed to lithium during labor. Hypothyroidism and diabetes can also occur in infants exposed to toxic levels of lithium. For this reason, close monitoring of lithium levels in the mother during labor is now routine (Yonkers, et al., 2004).

Levels of lithium in the blood may be affected by vomiting, salt intake, and illnesses that cause fevers. As pregnancy progresses, the kidneys eliminate lithium faster than usual, so the dose must typically be increased so that it remains at an effective level (Yonkers, et al., 2004). According to Yonkers and colleagues, it is important that pregnant women who use lithium stay hydrated; their doctors may consider giving them intravenous fluids if these women are in prolonged labor. They indicate that fetal anomalies resulting from first trimester exposure to lithium can be detected by prenatal screening using a high-resolution ultrasound examination and fetal echocardiography at weeks 16-18 of the pregnancy. This can help parents make decisions regarding pregnancy termination and interventions that the baby may need to undergo after delivery (Yonkers et al., 2004).

Anticonvulsants. Anticonvulsant medications, also referred to as antiepileptic drugs (AEDs), have been used to prevent seizures in people with epilepsy as well as depressive episodes of BD (Yonkers et al., 2004). A 2012 epigenetic study of 201 mothers with mental illnesses and/or epilepsy and their newborn babies examined the DNA methylation levels in the umbilical cord blood of newborns, including 53 infants exposed to various AEDs during pregnancy (Smith et al., 2012). Results of the study revealed a statistically significant correlation between an increased length of time that newborns were exposed to AEDs in utero and a decreased level of DNA methylation on certain DNA regions. DNA methylation is associated with genetic expression, which affects "fundamental developmental and regulatory processes" (Smith et al., 2012, p. 458). This study indicates that further research is warranted into the effects of AED exposure during pregnancy, as they may pose a danger of fetal malformations.

Guidelines for the treatment of women with BD advise those treated with antiepileptic (anticonvulsant) medications take 3-5mg of folic acid daily, to prevent neural tube defects in fetuses exposed to these medications (Viguera, 2007). This recommendation is based on the knowledge that the primary potential benefits of folic acid occur early in the prenatal period, often before a woman realizes she has conceived.

Divalproex (Depakote®) or valproic acid (Depakene®). It is well-documented that valproic acid is associated with the highest rate of major congenital malformations (6.2%-16%) of all medications used to treat BD (Nguyen, Sharma, & McIntyre, 2009). A recent review summarizing research on the risks of valproic acid indicated that congenital malformations associated with this medication include neural tube defects (such as spina bifida, 1%-5%, in which the backbone and spinal canal do not close before birth), hydrocephalus (a buildup of fluid inside the skull which leads to brain swelling), microcephaly (head size 2 standard deviations below expected size, which is associated with abnormal brain function and reduced life expectancy), heart defects, urogenital defects, and *fetal valproate syndrome* (i.e., physical traits including flat nasal bridge; epicanthal folds, skin folds which cover the inner corner of the eyelid; small upper lips, and a downward-turned mouth, which are consistently observed in fetuses exposed to valproate), and multiple other anomalies (Nguyen et al., 2009). The teratogenic effects of valproate are reported to be dose-dependent; a dose increase from 1400 mg daily or less to more than 1400 mg daily increased the risk for major congenital malformations from 5.5% to 34.5% in infants studied (Vajda & Eadie, 2005). Children exposed to valproate in the womb are significantly more likely to display significant decreases in IQ and require special education (Goldstein, Corbin, & Fung, 2000; Meador et al. as referened in Smith et al., 2012). In addition, exposure to valproate in utero is associated with an increased risk for symptoms and diagnosis of both attention deficit hyperactivity disorder and autistic spectrum disorders (Moore et al., 2000; Rasalam et al., 2005).

Carbamazepine (Tegretol®). A rate of 2.2%-7.9% of adverse events in fetuses has been reported after exposure to carbamazepine in the womb (Nguyen et al., 2009). The rate of spina bifida in carbamazepine-exposed fetuses (0.5%-1%) is 5-10 times higher than that of controls (Nguyen, Sharma, & McIntyre, 2009). Heart defects are estimated at two times the rate of controls, which is 1.5%-2%; while cleft lip and cleft palate are reported at five times the rate of controls (Nguyen et al., 2009). A higher incidence of birth defects was reported when carbamazepine was used in conjunction with valproate (Matalon, et al., 2002).

Lamotrigine (Lamictal®). The findings from an international lamotrigine pregnancy registry, which involved over 400 first-trimester exposures to lamotrigine alone revealed that the overall risk for major malformations is about 2.9%, whereas the baseline risk for major malformations in the general population is between 2% and 4% (Viguera, 2005). One study found an increased risk (5.4%) of major fetal anomalies among mothers who took lamotrigine during the first trimester at dosages greater than 200 mg daily, but this increased risk was not found in a larger study (Newport et al., 2008). Lamotrigine use is associated with a 10-24 times increased risk of oral clefts (e.g., cleft lip, cleft palate; 4-8.9 per 1000 births) than the general population (0.37 per 1000 births; Viguera et al., 2007). Pregnant women using lamotrigine may need to have their dosages increased due to the potential increase in metabolic clearance of the drug during pregnancy (Newport, et al., 2008).

In one study of 26 women with BD who either discontinued mood stabilizers (lithium, lamotrigine, or divalproex) or continued using lamotrigine during pregnancy, 30% of those who continued using lamotrigine relapsed versus 100% of those who discontinued using mood stabilizers. All of the women who relapsed while continuing lamotrigine treatment had depressive or mixed episodes, whereas 18.8% of new episodes without mood stabilizers were of the manic or hypomanic variety (Newport, et al., 2008). Those who continued using lamotrigine and relapsed had a much longer time before they experienced their first mood episode than those who discontinued mood stabilizer use (mean ± SD = 7.7 ± 7.4 versus 32.5 ± 13.2 weeks; Newport et al., 2008, p. 434).

Antipsychotics. Johnson et al. (2012) conducted a prospective, controlled study, which compared 309 mother-infant dyads 6 months postpartum. Infants had been exposed to antipsychotics, antidepressants, or no psychotropic medications in utero ($n =$ 22, 202, and 85, respectively.) They were administered a standardized test of posture, tone, reflexes, motor skills, and visual habituation. Results indicated that the infants of mothers who used antipsychotic medications during pregnancy showed significantly lower scores on this test than did those of mothers who used antidepressants or forewent medication during pregnancy. This study indicates that the safety of antipsychotic drug use should be further evaluated and that caution should be used when prescribing this type of medication.

Typical antipsychotics. Typical antipsychotic drugs have been used for decades, and more (albeit still limited) data on their safety is available than for mood stabilizers as a result (Stowe & Newport, 2007). Phenothiazines—including perphenazine (Trilafon®), chlorpromazine (Thorazine®) and prochlorperazine (Compazine®*)*—and butyrophenones (e.g., haloperidol, brand-name Haldol®) have historically been used to treat nausea, vomiting, and psychotic disorders during pregnancy; they are the drug classes with the most reproductive information available within this group (Stowe & Newport, 2007). While these drugs appear to be safe during pregnancy based on limited data, they are known to cause side effects in some women, which include tardive dyskinesia (a disorder that involves involuntary movements, especially of the lower face) and hyperprolactinemia (a disorder that causes some women to become infertile and produce breast milk in the absence of pregnancy; Minick & Atlas, 2007).

Atypical antipsychotics. There is limited data available on the safety of this group of drugs during pregnancy, but there is no conclusive evidence that they cause fetal malformations (Eberhard-Gran, Eskild, & Opjordsmoen, 2005). Eight cases of major congenital malformations were reported in association with risperidone (Risperdal®) exposure in utero (Nguyen et al., 2009). In this same literature review, the authors reported that increased risk of major congenital malformation was not found to be significantly associated with quetiapine (Seroquel®) use. Developmental delay has been preliminarily reported after in utero exposure to ziprasidone (Geodon®), although safety data regarding ziprasidone in humans is insufficient to warrant any conclusive results.

Olanzapine (Zyprexa®). Olanzapine is associated with weight gain and diabetes mellitus, both of which can negatively affect the outcome of the birth. Cases of cleft lip, encephalocele, and aqueductal stenosis have been documented in infants born to mothers who used olanzapine during their pregnancies. A 1% incidence of birth defects with the use of olanzapine was reported in one report (Goldstein et al., 2000). In one study, a 30.8% rate of neonatal intensive care admissions and low birth weights was reported for infants exposed to olanzapine in utero (Newport et al., 2007). Clozapine (Clozaril®) is also associated with weight gain and diabetes in mothers.

Medication use during the various stages of pregnancy.

The preconception stage. Viguera, Cohen, Bouffard, et al. (2002) suggested that those wanting to discontinue medication use during pregnancy should engage in a trial period long before they become pregnant, to give themselves and their doctors an idea of how they feel off of medication. Those who do well may take that as encouragement that they may at least try to forego medication during the first trimester of pregnancy and perhaps beyond. Those who have negative reactions will likely need to work with their physicians to figure out a medication regimen that they are both comfortable with (Viguera, Cohen, Baldessarini et al., 2002). The preconception stage is a good time for women with BD to empower themselves by learning about the teratogenic potential of various medications used to treat BD. Women should ensure that they have OB-GYNs who work productively with their psychiatrists or family physicians who oversee their psychotropic medications.

The prenatal stage. In a prospective observational study of 89 pregnant women with BD, 37% of those who continued using medication versus 85.5% of those who discontinued medication use had at least one recurrence of their mood disorder (Viguera et al., 2007). Most recurrences (74%) were depression or a mixed state rather than mania or hypomania. Risk in the first, second, and third trimesters was 47.2%, 31.9%, and 18.8%, respectively. Women who stopped using their mood stabilizers abruptly, that is, in 14 days or less, had a 50% risk of recurrence of mood episode during 2 weeks. Those who took longer to decrease their medication doses did not reach a 50% relapse rate until week 22 of pregnancy. Rapid discontinuation of medicine was much more likely with unplanned pregnancies (95.8% of unplanned versus 20.3% of planned pregnancies) (Viguera et al., 2007). Those who continued medication treatment met criteria for a mood episode for 8.8% of the time they were pregnant. Those who discontinued medication treatment met criteria for a mood episode 43.3% of the time they were pregnant.

The postpartum stage. The risk for postpartum BD relapse is estimated to be between 50% and 70% for those who do not take any medication as they approach delivery (Viguera, 2005). Five studies of lithium as a method of preventing postpartum bipolar mood episodes showed that women who restarted lithium regimens near their delivery dates reduced their risk of relapse from 50% to 10% (Viguera, 2005). Viguera recommended that her patients restart their bipolar medications at 36 weeks of pregnancy so that they are using therapeutic dosages by the time they deliver; she sometimes has patients use their medications again right after the first trimester because "we know that becoming ill during pregnancy is the strongest predictor for becoming ill postpartum" (Viguera, 2005, p. 3).

Lactation. Breast-fed infants have been found to have lower rates of gastrointestinal disease, atopic dermatitis, asthma, diabetes, lower respiratory tract diseases, otitis media, childhood leukemia, and sudden infant death syndrome; additionally, mothers who breast-feed their babies have a decreased risk of breast cancer, ovarian cancer, and maternal type II diabetes (Ip et al., 2007). Guidelines regarding the safety of psychotropic drugs during lactation are based on very limited data. The American Academy of Pediatrics (AAP, 2001) does not recommend lithium use during lactation because it is associated with increased rates of low muscle tone, heart murmur, lethargy, cyanosis (bluish skin discoloration caused by a lack of oxygen in the blood), and changes in electrocardiogram readings among infants. Carbamazepine and valproate are considered compatible with breastfeeding. However, the AAP reports that the effects on infants of using lamotrigine, chlorpromazine, haloperidol and clozapine during breastfeeding are unknown but might include therapeutic levels in infants' systems (associated with lamotrigine), declines in developmental scores (associated with haloperidol and chlorpromazine), and galactorrhea (spontaneous flow of milk from the breast) in mothers and drowsiness and lethargy in infants (associated with chlorpromazine; AAP, 2001).

One author noted that taking medication immediately after breast-feeding maximizes clearance before the next feeding and minimizes the amount present in the milk (Kacew, 1993). Other authods noted that medication should not be switched for breastfeeding because it exposes the child to more medications and to multiple medications for a period of time, due to the delay of neonatal clearance of the original drug (Stowe & Newport, 2007). Should a mother choose to breast-feed while taking psychotropic medication, her pediatrician should be informed so that the child can be monitored monthly; this will help ensure that the infant is healthy and meeting normal developmental milestones (Burt & Rasgon, 2004). Feeding an infant formula some of the time is a way to reduce infant exposure to drugs while still providing some breast-feeding benefits. Using the lowest possible dose to maintain psychiatric stability and just one medication is recommended also (Burt & Rasgon, 2004). However, using doses that are so low that they constitute ineffective treatment exposes the infant to medication needlessly (Burt et al., 2001).

Conclusions. Studies of medication use among women with BD typically have quite a few limitations, which are to be expected when conducting research with such a high-risk population. Random assignment to experimental and control groups is all but impossible due to human participant ethical rules. Small sample sizes are typically used due to the difficulty in finding willing subjects. There are many uncontrollable variables involved, due to the differing types and severity levels of BD, the need for individualized treatment plans (including many different medications and the use of multiple medications in combination). Sample populations may not be representative of the larger population because those who participate are usually those who have researched the topic more extensively and those who are receiving particularly high levels of medical care. Nonetheless, these studies provide valuable insight into an important topic that is difficult to research.

Summary. There is evidence that many psychiatric medications used to treat and prevent BD increase the risk of birth defects in infants exposed to them in the womb; there is also lack of evidence that other psychiatric drugs do not increase this risk (Yonkers et al., 2004). Viguera, Cohen, Baldessarini et al. (2002) suggested that women with BD wanting to discontinue medication use during pregnancy engage in a trial period long before they become pregnant to give themselves and their doctors an idea of how they feel off of medication. If they develop new mood episodes, women should work with their physicians to form a plan that utilizes the safest medications at the lowest therapeutic dosage (Yonkers et al., 2004). If they do not develop new mood episodes, they can then try to forgo their use during the first trimester, the period of time when the fetus is most susceptible to teratogens, and perhaps beyond (Viguera, 2007). Guidelines regarding the safety of psychotropic drugs during lactation are based on very limited data (The American Academy of Pediatrics, 2001). An informational resource written from the perspective of clinical psychology could clarify the complex issue of medication safety for women with BD and enable them to ask their physicians the questions they need answered in order to make informed decisions on the matter.

Psychosocial and Complementary Interventions for BD and their Relevance to Pregnancy

Given the known and unknown teratogenic risks of medications used to treat BD during pregnancy, women with the disorder would likely be interested in learning about alternatives to medication, such as behavioral, psychotherapeutic, and complementary interventions that would prevent mood episodes without posing harm to their unborn children. They may prefer to use both medication and nontraditional therapies in the hope that their BD will become more effectively controlled, or they may use add-on treatment strategies so that they will not need as much medication during and in the immediate aftermath of pregnancy. Due to the ethical problems inherent in conducting randomly controlled trials of pregnant women with BD, it would be extremely difficult to gather any direct evidence which would support the use of alternative treatments for BD during pregnancy. However, evidence that supports the use of alternative interventions for BD and depression among those who are not pregnant is available. In addition, some of these interventions have been tested on pregnant people who do not have BD. It can be conjectured that the treatments supported in these populations could potentially be helpful when applied to pregnant women with BD.

Psychosocial interventions for BD specific to pregnancy. Thus far, there exist no published resources from the perspective of mental health practitioners that delineate psychosocial interventions to treat BD during pregnancy. No controlled trials have been performed to assess the effect of nonpharmacological interventions on BD among postpartum women either (Burt, 2004). There are a few websites that briefly mention that psychotherapy may help treat BD during pregnancy, but that is the extent of the behavioral or complementary medicine advice given. Two books have been written on the topic of BD and pregnancy, and although neither of them focus on psychosocial interventions for the treatment of BD, women with BD might find them helpful in order to be better informed of the issues they may face while pregnant, which can help them plan their own pregnancies.

Bipolar and Pregnant: How to Manage and Succeed in Planning and Parenting While Living with Manic Depression is a first-person account of a woman with BD's experience of pregnancy (Finn, 2007). Some advice from experts, including a geneticist, psychologist, psychiatrist, and obstetrician, is included in the book. Finn's husband and mother's experience of having a pregnant, loved one with BD is included, too. The author described the great deal of planning she and her husband put into both of her pregnancies. She recommended journal writing as a means to monitor one's symptoms, and she recommended exercise as a stress-reliever. She also switched to a less stressful, part-time job in preparation for tapering off of her medications.

The book appears to be very useful to women with BD who are considering becoming pregnant because it not only conveys an idea of the issues that are important regarding BD and pregnancy, but it also provides advice from experts about how to avoid new mood episodes while maintaining the safety of the fetus. However, due to the highly variable nature of BD's presentation across individuals, a tool which provides information on the presentation of BD in a variety of women might provide a more realistic picture of what women with BD may expect during pregnancy. Also, the woman who wrote this book made the decision to go off of her medications, a decision that is contraindicated for women with a history of severe BD.

Bipolar and Pregnant provides a good deal of hope to women with BD because the author had a fairly good experience of pregnancy overall; she did not have to be hospitalized, nor did she experience severe symptoms. Another first-hand account of pregnancy from a woman with BD's perspective did not present such a pleasant picture: *Ride at Your Own Risk: A Guide for Pregnant Women with Bipolar Disorder and Their Families by Someone Who's Done It* (Bailey, 2008). This book described the emotionally tumultuous pregnancy of a woman who had poorly controlled BD who became pregnant. She was hospitalized or in day-treatment programs throughout much of her pregnancy. This book seems like it would be less useful for women with BD who are considering becoming pregnant because it did not provide many recommendations on how to avoid mood episodes. However, it was useful in the sense that it conveyed the painful emotions the author felt during pregnancy, and it was an honest account about the symptoms of BD she experienced. It is a cautionary story that makes the reader want to avoid unplanned pregnancies and work towards remission before becoming pregnant. The book also highlighted the importance of choosing the right clinicians to help one through the pregnancy process.

Psychotherapeutic interventions for the management of BD. Family-focused treatment, interpersonal and social rhythm therapy, cognitive-behavioral therapy, mindfulness-based cognitive therapy, dialectical behavior therapy, and MAPS (monitoring, assessing, preventing relapse, smart goal setting) group therapy are all psychotherapeutic interventions for the treatment of BD that have been supported with empirical evidence (Castle et al., 2007; Goldstein et al., 2007; Miklowitz et al., 2007; Wiliams et al., 2008). Although none of these interventions have been specifically tested on pregnant women with BD, they do stimulate ideas for how one might intervene with women with BD regarding pregnancy planning. These interventions are discussed in detail in this section.

Family-focused treatment. Family-focused treatment (FFT) for BD evolved from family psychoeducational models used to treat schizophrenia (Miklowitz & Goldstein, 1997). The treatment design is based on the finding that higher rates of family stress, as indicated by a person with BD's familial level of *expressed emotion* is linked to higher rates of bipolar relapse (Miklowitz, 2008). Expressed emotion is a measurable construct that represents the family's treatment of the individual with the disorder. Emotional reactions from family members that have been found to have an impact on relapse in individuals with BD (as well as schizophrenia) include critical comments, hostility, or emotional over-involvement with the family member (Miklowitz, 2008). FFT aims to reduce rates of expressed emotion in the families of those living with BD and to strengthen the social support of those living with BD.

FFT consists of 3 modules: *psychoeducation, communication enhancement training,* and *problem-solving skills*, which involve the client, as well as at least one family member, which is usually the spouse or parent. FFT is a manual-based treatment that consists of 21 sessions, which focus on helping the patient and their relatives meet the following six objectives: integrate the experiences associated with mood episodes in BD; accept the idea of a vulnerability to future episodes of BD; accept dependency on mood-stabilizing medications for symptom control; distinguish between the patient's personality and their BD; recognize and learn to cope with stressful life events that trigger BD recurrences; and re-establish functional relationships after a mood episode

(Miklowitz, 2008). FFT has not been utilized specifically on pregnant women who have bipolar disorder, or around pregnancy planning or postpartum issues. However, it appears to be potentially useful for this population, given the importance of family to both this treatment approach and pregnant women.

Randomized trials suggest that when combined with pharmacotherapy, FFT is one of the most efficacious psychotherapeutic interventions for the treatment of BD (Miklowitz et al., 2007). Miklowitz et al. (2003) conducted a randomized controlled trial of 101 adults with BD who were assigned to FFT plus pharmacotherapy ($n = 31$) or a less intensive crisis management intervention (CM) plus pharmacotherapy ($n = 70$). In order to be included in the study, subjects needed to have met *DSM-III* criteria for BD within the past 3 months. They also were required to be living with or having at least 4 hours of contact weekly with a caregiving family member, and they were excluded from the study if they had any alcohol or substance use disorders within the 6 months prior to the beginning of the study. Subjects' mood symptoms were assessed every 3 to 6 months for 2 years with the Schedule for Affective Disorders and Schizophrenia, Change Version (SADS-C). Medication compliance was assessed through subjects' self-report of inconsistency with medication, which was checked against reports by family members and physicians.

Results from this study indicated that over the 2-year trial, those in the FFT group had a three-fold higher rate of survival without BD relapse (52%) than did those in the CM group (17%). The FFT group also stayed well for an average of almost 5 months longer than the CM group (73.5 weeks vs. 53.2 weeks). The benefits of FFT extended beyond the 9 months of treatment. Subjects in the FFT group adhered to their medication regimen more than those in the CM group. There was no effect of drug adherence on subjects' depression scores at follow-up. However, those who were more adherent to their medications consistently had lower mania scores over time than their less adherent counterparts. Once drug adherence scores were covaried out, the main effect of psychosocial treatments on mania scores disappeared, suggesting that adherence mediated the effect of psychosocial interventions on mania symptoms. (In other words, psychosocial interventions caused individuals to be more adherent to their medications).

The authors of this study concluded that FFT plus pharmacotherapy reduces post-episode symptoms and increases drug adherence in people with BD. However, these conclusions may not be warranted because the study involved many confounding variables. For example, the number of sessions between the two groups differed greatly (21 sessions vs. 2 sessions plus crisis intervention). Because the FFT clinicians had more opportunities to observe subjects, it is possible that they were able to intervene when prodromal symptoms of relapse first appeared. Nevertheless, this study is important because it suggested that FFT is an effective way to drastically decrease the relapse rate in those with BD, in particular those who had recently had a mood episode. It also provided some evidence that psychosocial interventions are best used to prevent depressive symptoms rather than manic symptoms. If couples could learn more effective communication and problem-solving skills before they become pregnant, perhaps the number of stressful interactions could be reduced, lowering the risk of BD relapse during pregnancy and postpartum.

In another randomized trial of FFT versus individual psychotherapy, participants were 53 adults with BD, who had recently been hospitalized for a manic episode, and their families (Rea et al., 2003). All participants were taking medication at the time of the study, and they did not have chronic alcohol or substance abuse/dependence. Results of the study revealed that over the 1 year of treatment and 1 year of follow-up, the FFT group was less likely to be rehospitalized than the individual treatment group. The FFT group also had fewer total mood disorder relapses, although they were as likely to have a first relapse as the individual treatment group. Interestingly, the greatest effects of FFT were found after the treatment was complete during the post-treatment year of follow-up: 28% of FFT subjects relapsed versus 60% of subjects in the individualized treatment group. Additionally, only 12% of FFT subjects were hospitalized during this time period compared to 60% of subjects in the individualized treatment group. This finding demonstrates the efficacy of FFT because it suggests that clients and their families needed to learn all of the information provided by FFT before they could fully benefit from it.

Authors of the study concluded that FFT is useful as an adjunct to pharmacotherapy for the prevention of BD relapse and hospitalization. It is possible that this conclusion is erroneous because it is based on a comparison of two groups, which not only differed by treatment approach, but which also differed by number of therapists (2 for FFT vs. 1 for individualized treatment) and session length (60 minutes for FFT vs. 30 minutes for individualized treatment). Nonetheless, this study was of a better design than the one mentioned previously because therapist-client contact was of equal in terms of duration (9 months) and number of sessions (21). Thus, group differences cannot be attributed to better monitoring of clients' new symptoms by clinicians, which was not the case in the previous study mentioned. Another weakness of the study is that it did not include people whose most recent episode was of a depressed, hypomanic, or mixed nature; it also excluded people in partial or full remission. Therefore, it is unknown if results would generalize to these populations. If FFT is to be used for the prevention of bipolar relapse and hospitalization in pregnant women, the full treatment should be completed approximately 1 year before the woman conceives so that it can be of maximum benefit to these women.

The largest study to date comparing psychosocial adjuncts to pharmacotherapy was the systematic treatment enhancement program for bipolar disorder (STEP-BD; Miklowitz et al., 2007). Participants were 152 adults with either bipolar I disorder ($n = 105$) or bipolar II disorder ($n = 47$), who were experiencing a current major depressive episode. Baseline scores were measured by the Longitudinal Interval Follow-Up Evaluation-Range of Impaired Functioning Tool (LIFE-RIFT). Those who had a substance misuse disorder (besides nicotine) were excluded. Subjects were randomly assigned to thirty 1-hour sessions (21 weekly and 9 biweekly) of intensive psychosocial treatment in the form of FFT ($n = 13$), cognitive-behavioral therapy (CBT; $n = 38$), or interpersonal and social rhythm therapy ($n = 33$), or three 1-hour sessions of collaborative care treatment over 6 weeks ($n = 68$). Stratification of variables was performed based on bipolar I or bipolar II status, as well as that of 15 study sites at which the treatment was conducted. At entry and then every 3 months over the 9-month treatment period, subjects' levels of depression and role functioning were assessed with the Montgomery-Asberg Depression Rating Scale and LIFE-RIFT, respectively. The LIFE-RIFT assesses 4 domains: relationships, satisfaction, work/role performance, and recreational activities/hobbies. The authors sought to determine whether intensive psychosocial interventions plus pharmacotherapy would improve the vocational or social functioning of people with BD and whether these improvements would be independent of depression severity.

Results of the study showed that intensive psychotherapy improved total functioning, relationship functioning, and life satisfaction scores beyond the level of improvements expected from changes in depressed mood. Psychosocial interventions did not increase subjects' work/role functioning or recreation scores during the 9-month period. The authors concluded that intensive psychotherapy improves the life satisfaction and relationship functioning of people with BD. These conclusions seem to be warranted based on the data, but this study has some of the same flaws as the two studies of FFT mentioned above: differing amounts of client-therapist contact between control and experimental groups and overly specific mood episode recruitment criteria that make it difficult to generalize to other people with BD who may have recently experienced a mood episode of a different type. The study also excluded those with substance abuse problems, which may have excluded those with severe BD. Nevertheless, the results hold some promise for pregnant women with BD. Relationship functioning and life satisfaction are arguably the two domains that have the greatest impact on the stress levels of pregnant women. The findings of the study suggests that perhaps these areas of functioning could both be improved for pregnant women with BD via intensive psychotherapeutic interventions.

Interpersonal and social rhythm therapy. The social *zeitgeber* (i.e., time-giver) hypothesis posits that unstable or disrupted daily routines lead to circadian rhythm instability and to mood episodes in vulnerable individuals (Frank, 2005). It has been demonstrated that in addition to medication nonadherence and stressful life events, disruptions in daily routines (trans-Atlantic travel, working a night shift, becoming a mother) are indeed associated with the onset of depression and especially mania (Malkoff-Schwartz et al., 2000; Malkoff-Schwartz et al., 1998). Interpersonal and social rhythm therapy (IPSRT) aims to help those with BD develop more regular daily and nightly routines; these "social rhythms" include sleeping, waking, eating, socializing (Frank, 2007). This is accomplished by tracking sleep/wake cycles and daily routines and keeping routines despite the occurrence of events that would normally disrupt them. IPSRT also helps individuals with BD to resolve grief for the lost "healthy self" and to improve their interpersonal relationships (Frank, 2005).

To date, two randomized, controlled trials of IPSRT have been conducted. The first trial of IPSRT's effectiveness was conducted in the context of the STEP-BD study mentioned previously. Results indicated that as an adjunct to medication, IPSRT was one of the three intensive psychosocial treatments that was found to improve total functioning, relationship functioning, and life satisfaction over 9 months when compared to collaborative care (Miklowitz, et al., 2007). The second study of the efficacy of IPSRT for BD compared IPSRT to intensive clinical management (ICM), an adaptation of the clinical management strategy used in the National Institute of Mental Health Treatment of Depression Collaborative Research Program, also as an adjunct to pharmacotherapy.

The study involved 175 adult outpatients diagnosed with either bipolar I disorder or schizoaffective disorder, manic type. All subjects were in the acute phase of their third or greater lifetime depressive, manic, or mixed episode (Frank, 2005). Exclusion criteria included current rapid cycling, chronic substance abuse, pregnancy, uncontrolled medical illness that would preclude pharmacotherapy, and having borderline or antisocial personality, active bulimia, or anorexia. The participants were assigned to one of four treatment strategies: acute and maintenance IPSRT, acute and maintenance ICM, acute IPSRT followed by maintenance ICM, or acute ICM followed by maintenance IPSRT. The Research Diagnostic Criteria was used to assess the presence of an affective episode in subjects both at study entrance and time of recurrence. The Hamilton Depression Rating Scale and the Bech-Rafaelsen Mania Scale were used to determine severity of depression and mania. The Social Rhythm Metric I (SRM I), a measure of the regularity of daily routines, was completed by subjects receiving ICM. The Social Rhythm Metric II (SRM II), an adaptation of the SRM I designed to help participants increase the regularity of their routines, was completed by those receiving IPSRT.

Results of this study revealed that those who received IPSRT in the acute phase of treatment had more regular daily routines, as indicated by their higher SRM scores. They also survived longer on average without a new mood episode than those who received ICM in the acute phase of treatment and were also more likely to remain well for the full 2 years of the study's preventive maintenance phase. There were no differences in medication adherence across the four groups. The authors concluded that the finding that IPSRT works best when initiated during the acute phase of illness rather than the maintenance phase may be explained by ill subjects having more motivation than well subjects to introduce the difficult lifestyle changes that IPSRT demands.

IPSRT sessions were about 25 minutes longer than ICM sessions; hence, it is possible that the results could be influenced by subjects having more support in general, rather than more of a specific type of support. However, this does not seem likely given that the IPSRT benefits appeared to be mediated by increased social rhythm stability. Also, subjects with more medical problems actually benefited more from the shorter ICM sessions, which may be explained by the greater focus of ICM on physical symptoms. Thus, the authors' conclusions appear to be warranted by the data. Pregnancy could be a time when more somatically focused treatments, such as ICM, would be more helpful than IPSRT. However, it is likely that pregnant women with BD would be highly motivated to enact the changes recommended by IPSRT, so this treatment may prove helpful to this population nevertheless.

Cognitive-behavioral therapy. Although cognitive-behavioral therapy (CBT) for the treatment of BD does involve psychoeducation, its main focus is on implementing self-monitoring strategies so that those with BD are able to recognize the effect that their emotions, thoughts, and behaviors have on their illness (Basco, 1996). Cognitive restructuring exercises and step-wise behavioral assignments are utilized in order to improve coping skills. More randomized trials of the effectiveness of CBT for the treatment of BD have been conducted than for any other psychotherapeutic approach to this disorder. Different models of CBT interventions, such as schema-focused or psychoeducation with CBT added to it, have been used by different investigators. Studies have differed in their emphases as well: Some focused on CBT for the prevention of relapse in individuals not experiencing currently mood episodes, while others have focused on CBT for individuals in the midst of acute mood episodes. Participant characteristics have also varied tremendously across studies; some included only individuals whose illness was in remission, while others included syndromally or subsyndromally ill individuals (Miklowitz, 2009). Some studies excluded those with comorbid substance abuse, Axis 1, or personality disorders, while others did not. Due to the various differences across studies, inconsistent cross-trial conclusions have been reported. However, meta-analyses indicate that CBT is an important part of outpatient care of those with BD, with the most profound benefits being found for the prevention of depressive relapse.

Lam et al. (2003) sought to determine whether cognitive therapy (CT) plus mood stabilizers and regular psychiatric follow-up was more effective in preventing relapse than mood stabilizers plus regular psychiatric follow-up in a subgroup of people with BD who were vulnerable to relapse. One hundred and three adults with recurrent episodes of bipolar I disorder (defined as either 2 mood episodes in the last 2 years or 3 mood episodes in the last 5 years) who were not actively suicidal and did not currently meet criteria for a bipolar episode or substance abuse disorder were randomly assigned to either a control group or a group that received on average 14 CT sessions. Subjects were only included in the study if they had a Beck Depression Inventory (BDI) score lower than 30 and a Bech-Rafaelsen Mania Rating Scale (MRS) score lower than 9.

At the beginning of the study, subjects were administered the Structured Clinical Interview for *DSM-IV* (SCID-I), the Medical Research Council Social Performance Schedule, and the Coping with Prodromes Interview. At 6- and 12-month follow-up, independent assessors blind to subjects' group status assessed subjects with the SCID-I to determine whether or not they had relapsed (i.e., met criteria for a major depressive, manic, or hypomanic mood episode). At 1-month intervals, the BDI Internal State Scale (ISS) and the Beck Hopelessness Scale (BHS) were administered to assess mood fluctuations; the control subscale of the Dysfunctional Attitudes Scale (Short Version) (DAS-SV) was also used to identify dysfunctional attitudes of extreme striving. Medication compliance was assessed every 6 months by report from participants' psychiatric service staff who had the most contact with them. The Medication Compliance Questionnaire was also completed monthly by participants. Every 6 months, participants' relatives in closest contact with them were interviewed in order to obtain information on participants' social functioning. Results of the study indicated that during the 12 months of the study, those in the CT group had significantly fewer bipolar episodes (43.8% vs. 75%), days in a bipolar episode (26.6 ± 46.0 vs. 88.4 ± 108.9), and number of admissions to a hospital for a bipolar episode (14.6% vs. 33.3%). The CT group also had significantly higher social functioning, significantly less fluctuation in manic symptoms, and showed less mood symptoms on the monthly mood questionnaires. They were also better at coping with manic prodromal symptoms at 12 months. Results from this study and those mentioned earlier in this section provide evidence that CT and CBT may be helpful in preventing bipolar relapses. Perhaps it would also be helpful in preventing relapses in pregnant women with BD.

Mindfulness-based cognitive therapy. Mindfulness-based cognitive therapy (MBCT) integrates mindfulness-based meditative practices with CT (Deckersbach et al., 2012). Its goal is to help people disengage from negative thought patterns by becoming aware of and accepting them as passing events rather than focusing on them in an attempt to change them; this helps people to avoid ruminating on their negative thoughts, which can lead to a downward spiral into depression. MBCT was originally developed as a treatment for recurrent depression. Its utility as an adjunctive treatment for BD has recently been studied.

Williams et al. (2008) analyzed data from a pilot study of MBCT for adults with remitted unipolar and bipolar disorders who had a history of suicidality. Treatment was implemented via groups that met for 2 hours weekly for 8 weeks, plus a full day of meditation following the 6th week of the study. In addition to attending the group, participants were asked to spend 45 minutes 6 days per week completing homework, which included meditating and observing their thoughts, feelings, and bodily sensations. They were instructed to continue taking their medication and/or utilizing outpatient services as usual. Fourteen adults with BD completed the study; they were equally divided among the treatment group and wait list groups. The BDI and BAI were used to assess treatment efficacy. Results indicated that anxiety and depressive symptoms significantly decreased from pretreatment to posttreatment among those diagnosed with BD who were in the treatment group.

Williams et al. (2008) concluded that MBCT showed an immediate reduction in symptoms of anxiety and depression among those diagnosed with BD who exhibited suicidal ideation or behaviors, although the power of the results was limited due to the small sample size. They noted that anxiety has a high rate of co-morbidity with BD (64%), and it is associated with poorer outcome among those diagnosed with BD (Sasson et al. and Simon et al. as cited in Williams et al, 2008). Thus, they expressed a belief that MBCT could hold promise as a treatment for BD, and further studies of its effectiveness may be warranted. These conclusions seem justified. It is important to note, however, that this study did not assess medication use or symptoms of mania or hypomania. The results of this study suggest that MBCT could potentially be helpful for pregnant women with BD, including those who experience anxiety or suicidality.

Deckersbach et al. (2012) conducted an open trial of twelve 120-minute, weekly group MBCT sessions in order to determine if they would improve the residual mood symptoms of the 10 adults diagnosed with nonremitted bipolar I or II. All but one participant were taking psychotropic medication to manage their BD. The HAM-D, YMRS, Five-Factor Mindfulness Questionnaire (FFMQ), Penn State Worry Questionnaire (PSWQ), Response Style Questionnaire (RSQ), Emotion Reactivity Scale (ERS), Adult ADHD Self-Report Scale (ASRS1.1), Clinical Positive Affect Scale (CPAS), the PWBS, and the LIFE-RIFT were used to assess symptoms of BD, general psychological well-being, psychosocial functioning, rumination, attention, and mindfulness skills. Results indicated that at posttreatment, participants generally reported increased mindfulness, lower residual depressive and hypomanic/manic symptoms and attention problems, and increased emotion-regulation skills, psychological well-being, positive affect, and psychosocial functioning. One participant reported experiencing a hypomanic episode 3 months after treatment. It is important to note that most improvements were not fully maintained 3 months posttreatment, which suggests that booster sessions may be warranted. Results indicated that emotion regulation and interpersonal relationships continued to improve from pretreatment through the follow-up period.

The authors of this pilot study concluded that MBCT can be utilized successfully with people with nonremitted BD; however, they noted that their results cannot be generalized to all people with BD due to the small sample size and lack of a randomized control group. The authors' conclusions seem warranted. This study provides further evidence that MBCT could potentially be a means of managing residual symptoms of BD. It seems to be a fairly safe option that could help pregnant women with BD manage their moods.

Dialectical behavior therapy. Dialectical behavior therapy (DBT) is an efficacious treatment for suicidal behavior and borderline personality disorder (BPD) that evolved from CBT (Linehan, et al., 2006). DBT focuses on the implementation of skills related to mindfulness, distress tolerance, emotion regulation, and interpersonal effectiveness (Van Dijk, 2009). BD has many symptoms in common with BPD, including impulsivity, difficulty regulating emotions, unstable relationships and unhealthy or self-destructive coping skills. Because of these similarities, it has been hypothesized that DBT would also be an effective treatment for BD (Van Dijk, 2009).

Van Dijk, Jeffrey, and Katz (2013) conducted a pilot randomized, controlled trial of the effectiveness of a 12-week program of 90-minute psychoeducational groups which taught DBT skills, mindfulness techniques, and general psychoeducation about BD to adults diagnosed with BD-I or BD-II. Twenty-six adults participated, half of whom were randomized to a wait-list control group. Those who participated in the experimental group were hospitalized less frequently for mental health related issues and reported less depressive symptoms than those in the control group. The results from this study provides preliminary evidence that DBT could potentially be useful for the treatment of BD in adults; however, further studies of its effectiveness with larger sample sizes are warranted before stronger conclusions can be drawn.

Goldstein et al. (2007) conducted a preliminary study of the effectiveness of DBT as an adjunct to medication for the treatment of BD in adolescents. Ten individuals aged

14-18 years old who had been diagnosed with Bipolar I, II, or not otherwise specified (NOS) with an acute manic, mixed, or depressive episode in the 3 months preceding the study participated. The Schedule for Affective Disorders (SAD) and Schizophrenia for School-Age Children-Present Depression Rating Scale (K-SADS-P-DRS), K-SADS Mania Rating Scale (MRS), and the Modified Scale for Suicidal Ideation (MSSI) were used to evaluate subjects' symptoms at baseline and every 3 months during the year-long study. Results of the study indicated that from pre- to post-treatment, subjects had significant improvements in suicidality, nonsuicidal self-injurious behavior, depressive symptoms, and emotional dysregulation. The authors concluded that because there was no comparison group, these improvements could not be contributed to DBT. Based on the data, this conclusion appears to be warranted. Although the trial did not provide definitive evidence of DBT's efficacy for the treatment of adolescents with BD, it did provide a glimpse at its potential. As there is no empirical evidence of DBT's efficacy in treating pregnant women with BD, its use with this population should be approached with caution.

MAPS (monitoring, assessing, preventing relapse, smart goal setting) group therapy. Castle et al. (2010) developed a psychoeducational group treatment manual for adults diagnosed with BD. This program includes: "monitoring mood and activities (M), assessing prodromes (A), preventing or reducing relapse (P) and setting Specific, Measurable, Achievable, Realistic, Time-Framed (SMART) goals (S), and is known by the acronym MAPS" (p. 384). They conducted a randomized, controlled trial of MAPS plus treatment as usual with 84 adults diagnosed with BD type I, II, or NOS who were receiving treatment from either a general practitioner or psychiatrist. Exclusion criteria included being diagnosed with a developmental disability or being in the midst of an acute mood episode during recruitment. The treatment group attended 12 weekly 90-minute psychoeducational group sessions plus 3 monthly booster sessions. They were also provided with workbooks, informational handbooks, and pocket-sized journals in which they were instructed to record their medication use and side effects, symptoms, relapse prevention plans, and negative thinking patterns, and then share them with their treatment team and key support persons (Castle et al., 2007). Researchers telephoned the participants weekly to remind them of the next group and answer any questions participants had about homework assignments. Participants in the control group received treatment as usual plus weekly telephone calls from the researchers. The Montgomery-Asberg Depression Rating Scale (MADRS) and the YMRS were used to assess rates of relapse pre- and post-treatment.

Results indicated that participants in the treatment group were significantly less likely to experience a mood episode during treatment and up to a year after treatment began. They also spent significantly fewer days unwell compared to the control group. The authors concluded that MAPS reduces the risk of relapse in those diagnosed with BD. This conclusion should be interpreted with caution given that the participants were not blind to which experimental group they were in. Participants assigned to the control group did not participate in a group of any kind. Overall, this study provides some evidence that MAPS group psychoeducation can be helpful in preventing relapse among people diagnosed with BD. It is possible that some of the interventions used in MAPS may also be helpful for the prevention of mood episodes among pregnant women diagnosed with BD.

Complementary, alternative, and behavioral approaches for the treatment of BD. The complementary and alternative medicine interventions of dark therapy, light therapy, electroconvulsive therapy, transcranial magnetic stimulation and nutrition therapy, as well as the behavioral interventions of exercise, yoga, mindfulness, and meditation are mentioned briefly in this section. Besides electroconvulsive therapy, none of these interventions have been tested on pregnant women with BD.

Dark therapy. Dark therapy (DT) is based on the hypothesis that unmonitored exposure to artificial light and sleep disruption due to environmental stimuli could trigger mood episodes in people with BD, while a strict control of the sleep-wake cycle and light-dark rhythms could act as a mood stabilizer. DT is a regimen of 14 hours of enforced darkness and rest in a sound-proof, light-sealed room from 6pm to 8am (14 hours) each night for 3 consecutive days. It has shown to have promise as an adjunctive treatment to medication for bipolar mania and rapid-cycling bipolar disorder (Barbini et al., 2005; Wehr et al., 1998; Wirz-Justice et al., 1999). DT was tested on 16 inpatients with BD affected by manic episodes at the time of the study (Barbini et al., 2005). These individuals also received therapy as usual (TAU), which included drug treatment. They were matched with other manic, bipolar inpatients for age, sex, age of onset, duration of current episode, and number of previous illness episodes. The control group also received TAU, but they were only required to stay in their rooms from 10 pm to 6 am. Severity of mania was rated on the Young Mania Rating Scale (YMRS) at baseline and every morning afterward.

Results of the study indicated that those exposed to DT who had been manic for less than 2 weeks had markedly better outcomes than the controls and those exposed to

DT who had been manic longer than 2 weeks. They slept an average of 5 hours more per night than the manic participants who were not exposed to DT. Their scores on the YMRS decreased much more quickly than those of the controls, and the length of time they had to stay in the hospital was shorter by 8.9 days. Additionally, they left the hospital with fewer antimanic medications and lower doses of those medications. There were no differences between the experimental and control groups for individuals who had been manic longer than 2 weeks. The authors of the study concluded that control of environmental stimuli and interventions that focus on the circadian rhythm can be a useful add-on for the treatment of acute mania in a hospital setting. Given the small sample size and lack of randomization, these conclusions seem a bit tenuous. Nonetheless, DT could prove beneficial to pregnant and postpartum women with BD experiencing mania because it could help them recover more quickly and with less medication.

Light therapy. Bright light therapy was first developed as a treatment for seasonal affective disorder (SAD). Since then, studies have shown that it is also effective in treating nonseasonal depression and bipolar depression (Sit et al., 2007). Light therapy involves the use of a *light box,* which emits differing amounts of ultraviolet-blocked white light. Light therapy's effectiveness and side effects depend on the time of day it is administered (typically early morning or midday), as well as the dose of light emitted. Variables affecting light dose include the duration of light exposure, distance from the light box, and intensity of emitted light. Eyestrain, headache, agitation, and nausea are the most commonly reported side effects. Mania, hypomania, insomnia, and suicidality have occurred in some people after beginning light therapy.

Sit et al. (2007) conducted a preliminary study of 9 women with nonseasonal, type I or II BD experiencing a depressive episode. Those taking herbs, beta blockers, or medication for an uncontrolled medical illness, as well as those with uncontrolled thyroid disease, generalized anxiety disorder, current psychosis, substance abuse within the last 6 months, or those who made a suicide attempt within the past 3 months were excluded from the study. The SCID-IV was used to verify diagnoses. The Structured Interview Guide for the Hamilton Depression Scale with Atypical Depression Supplement (SIGH-ADS) and the Mania Rating Scale (MRS) were used to assess mood severity. All participants were required to have taken at least one antimanic medication at a stable dose for 4 weeks prior to the study's beginning and to have continued to do so throughout the duration of the study. For the first 2 weeks of the 8-week study, subjects were exposed to 50 lux (dim) red light, which was used as a placebo. During the following 2 weeks, they were exposed to 7,000 lux (bright) light therapy for 15 minutes daily. During the next 2 weeks their exposure was extended to 30 minutes daily and during the last 2 weeks they received light therapy for 45 minutes daily. Four participants received morning light and five participants received midday (12 pm-2 pm) light.

Results of the study indicated that three of the four subjects exposed to morning light therapy developed mixed episodes. The fourth subject in this treatment group recovered fully and remained well. Of those receiving midday light therapy, 2 recovered fully and 2 showed improvements but needed an increased light dose to fully recover. One woman remained depressed despite receiving 45 minutes of midday light therapy daily; however, once her regimen was changed to 30 minutes daily of morning light, she, too, recovered fully. The study's authors concluded that women with BD are very sensitive to morning bright light therapy, and that they are at great risk of developing mixed episodes if treated with it. Instead, those suffering from bipolar depression should start by receiving 15 minutes of midday light therapy daily. Results of the study also indicated that three of the nine subjects developed vaginal bleeding once they began light therapy, although they had no underlying disorder that could explain its cause. The authors posited that light therapy's effects on the hypothalamic-pituitary-ovarian axis may have caused disruptions in these subjects' menstrual cycles.

The authors' conclusions appear to be warranted based on the limited data. With only nine participants, results of this study cannot be generalized to all women suffering from bipolar depression. Exclusion criteria were numerous and likely made the sample even less representative. Nonetheless, midday bright light therapy may prove to be quite useful for the treatment of bipolar depression during pregnancy if larger studies replicate these findings and prove that it is nonteratogenic. Given bright light therapy's demonstrated effects on the menstrual cycles and reproductive hormones of some of the women studied, special attention should be paid to its potential effects on the reproductive hormones of pregnant women in order to ensure its safety for this population (Danilenko & Samoilova, 2007). Pregnant women who receive light therapy should have someone help them identify prodromal mood symptoms to ensure that should they develop, light therapy can be discontinued immediately.

Electroconvulsive therapy. Anderson and Reti (2009) conducted a comprehensive review of the literature regarding the use of electroconvulsive therapy (ECT) during pregnancy from 1942 to 2007. They excluded articles that had not been written in English or translated into English. They found 339 articles on the subject.

Mothers included in the review had a variety of psychiatric illnesses, including BD ($n = 7$), major depressive disorder (MDD; $n = 37$), schizophrenia ($n = 18$), schizoaffective disorder ($n = 3$), undefined psychosis ($n = 3$); 271 of the cases reported did not state the mother's diagnosis. Pregnant women who underwent ECT and experienced full or partial remission included 85.7% of those with BD (6 out of 7), 83.8% of those with MDD (31 out of 37), and 100% of those with schizoaffective disorder (3 out of 3.) Of the 339 cases reviewed, fetal or neonatal abnormalities were reported in 25 of them, including 11 deaths; however, most of these abnormalities were not believed to be the result of ECT. The review's authors concluded that

> when likely non-ECT-related complications are excluded, the total number of fetal or neonatal abnormalities possibly related to ECT is 11, being eight cases of transient fetal arrhythmias, one fetal death secondary to grand mal seizure, one miscarriage in the first trimester 24 hours post ECT, and one case of multiple cortical and deep white matter infarctions after multiple ECT courses in the pregnant mother. (p. 239)

Of the 339 cases, 20 mothers experienced pregnancy complications themselves. Eighteen of these complications—which included uterine contractions and/or preterm labor ($n = 9$), vaginal bleeding ($n = 2$), grand mal seizure ($n = 1$), blood in the urine ($n = 1$), abdominal pain ($n = 1$), and placental abruption, a condition in which the placental lining separates from the mother's uterus before the baby is born ($n = 1$) —were thought to be at least partially related to ECT. Four of these cases also involved neonatal complications, as described previously. Side effects of ECT that can occur in the general population and were found to worsen with continuing treatment of pregnant women included confusion, memory loss, headaches, and muscle soreness.

The authors of this literature review concluded that the available data suggests ECT is efficacious during pregnancy and presents low risks to both the woman and child; they suggested that it should be considered in pregnant women with severe mental illness symptoms, such as psychotic symptoms, strong suicidal urges, or catatonia. Anderson and Reti (2009) acknowledged that a main limitation of this review was reporting biases. Normal or uneventful outcomes of ECT were much less likely to be reported in the literature than those which resulted in adverse or unusual outcomes. Another limitation of this literature review is that the results did not distinguish whether or not the mothers took psychotropic medications while they received ECT; thus, it is impossible to determine whether the treatment efficacy or adverse effects are due to ECT or medication.

Anderson and Reti (2009) noted that data on long-term effects of ECT on children whose mothers received the treatment are sparse. Data are available regarding 39 children ages 6 months to 19 years whose mothers received ECT while pregnant with them. All of the children were found to be defect-free, although two of them were described as "mentally deficient" (Andersson & Reti, 2009, p. 240). Richards (2007) stated that there is not enough data available to support the position of the American Psychiatric Association that ECT has low risk during each trimester of pregnancy. He stated that the rarity of ECT's use during pregnancy precludes it from being tested in a controlled trial with enough participants to demonstrate statistical significance. Although data available regarding the use of ECT for the treatment of BD during pregnancy is not strong, they do suggest that ECT may be a useful alternative treatment for this population should medication prove ineffective.

Transcranial magnetic stimulation. Transcranial magnetic stimulation (TMS) is a noninvasive intervention that can be used to either excite or inhibit certain areas of the brain, depending on whether repetitive stimulation is applied at high or low frequencies. The efficacy of TMS for treating depression, including bipolar depression, was evaluated in a 2001 Cochrane literature review. Results of the 16 studies included that were deemed to have adequately randomized control groups revealed "no strong evidence for a possible efficacy of transcranial magnetic stimulation for the treatment of depression, although these results do not exclude the possibility of benefit" (Rodriguez-Martin et al., 2001, p. 9).

Praharaj, Ram, and Arora (2009) conducted a single-blind, randomized controlled trial of high frequency (rapid) suprathreshold rTMS of the right prefrontal cortex compared to sham stimulation on 41 adult men and women with BD who were experiencing mania. Participants had been either *drug-naïve* or drug-free for at least the 2 months prior to the study's beginning. Eighty-five percent of the participants were male and 97.56% of participants (all but one) were experiencing mood-congruent psychotic symptoms. Subjects with history of drug abuse, epilepsy, significant head injury or neurosurgical procedure, those with current comorbid psychiatric or neurological illnesses, those with pacemakers or metal parts in their bodies, and those who had received ECT in the previous 6 months were excluded from the study. All participants began taking medication as soon as they entered the hospital where the trial took place. Those in the active group ($n = 21$) received 10 consecutive days of rTMS after undergoing a week of drug therapy. After one week of drug therapy, control group members ($n = 20$) received 10 consecutive days of rTMS with one wing of the coil tilted at a 45 degree angle to the head, which causes scalp sensations but does not produce the motor evoked potentials thought to be responsible for therapeutic effects. The Young Mania Rating Scale (YMRS) and Clinical Global Impression (CGI) were used to assess mania at baseline and after the 5th and 10th sessions of rTMS.

Both YMRS and CGI scores of those in the active group showed a small but statistically significantly decrease from pre- to post-treatment (mean YMRS score decreased from 20.85 ± 5.21 to 5.76 ± 3.26; mean CGI score decreased from 4.19 ± 0.60 to 2.42 ± 0.59) compared to the scores of those in the control group (mean YMRS score decreased from 19.35 ± 7.32 to 11.05 ± 6.86; mean CGI score decreased from 4.20 ± 0.76 to 3.10 ± 1.00.) The effect sizes for decreases in YMRS and CGI scores accounted for 6.2% and 1.44% of the total variance, respectively. All of the participants receiving active treatment reached remission versus 65% of those in the control group. One patient receiving active treatment developed depression during the study. Pain upon stimulation that improved on its own after the session was over was the most common complaint of those receiving active rTMS treatment; some participants in this group also reported headaches that lasted up to four hours (28.57%) and anxiety which decreased after reassurance (25%). The authors concluded that rapid supra-threshold right prefrontal rTMS was well tolerated and found to be effective as an adjunctive therapy to medication for the treatment of bipolar mania. Given the small sample size, lack of double-blinding, and stringent exclusionary criteria, this conclusion is not well-substantiated by the data. Also, the effect sizes were so small that rTMS methods would probably need to be further refined and demonstrate larger improvements in manic symptoms before its widespread use would be clinically indicated.

There are no large-scale studies of the safety of TMS during pregnancy. Zhang and Hu (2009) report administering repetitive TMS (rTMS) to three women in the early stages of pregnancy who were experiencing depression. All three women showed a significant reduction in depressive symptoms and birthed healthy babies who remained healthy throughout the 6-month post-treatment phase. Although these three cases did not demonstrate adverse effects, they do not provide any conclusive evidence for or against the safety or efficacy of TMS for BD during pregnancy, due to the very small sample size and lack of a randomized control group. Long-term effects were not examined in the mothers or infants. The report did not explicitly state whether or not the mothers were using antidepressant drugs concurrently with rTMS. Further research must be done on the matter before any conclusions can be drawn. For now, pregnant women with BD do not have much evidence upon which to base their decision to use or not use TMS. There is no convincing evidence that it is harmful to the mother or infant; nor is there convincing evidence that it is a safe or effective treatment for affective episode symptoms.

Nutrition therapy. There is a great deal of controversy regarding whether or not taking vitamin, mineral, fatty acid, amino acid, and botanical supplements ("nutritional therapy") may constitute an effective monotherapy or adjunctive treatment for BD.

Research on the subject has been around for decades but not many conclusions have been reached, seemingly due to lack of funding and lack of randomized controlled trials of high quality (Lakhan & Vieira, 2008).

EMPowerplus. A few case reports and uncontrolled trials suggest that a micronutrient supplement called EMPowerplus (EMP+) may be effective as a stand-alone treatment for children who have BD (Frazier et al., 2009). This 36-ingredient supplement manufactured by Truehope Nutritional Support Limited was the focus of a study of adults who claimed to have been diagnosed with BD (Gately & Kaplan, 2009). The manufacturers of the EMP+ formulation encourage their clients with psychiatric illnesses to complete an unvalidated self-report measure of mood symptoms they call the "Self-Monitoring Form" and mail it to them. Data from these forms were used as the basis for the study's results. Only subjects without co-morbid psychiatric diagnoses who reported symptoms 60 times or more over 6 months were included; the final sample consisted of 358 adults. Eighty-one percent of the study's participants were taking prescription medications commonly used to treat mood disorders.

The study's results indicated that use of the EMPowerplus micronutrient supplement was associated with a 41% decrease in mean symptom severity from baseline at 3 months and a 45% decrease at 6 months. The authors concluded that further research on EMP+ is warranted. This conclusion may be true. However, the study itself does not lend much empirical support for this conclusion because of the unvalidated outcome measure, lack of a control group, and large amount of self-selection bias that marred the study's design. Simply tracking ones' mood symptoms daily could have improved participants' mood symptom severity; it is a key strategy in many of the psychotherapeutic methods of treating BD (Basco, 1996; Frank, 2007). It would have been interesting to compare the rates of symptom severity with a placebo-controlled group that took psychiatric medications if they wanted to and completed a daily mood-tracking tool.

This study was not particularly helpful to pregnant women with BD because the weak study design precluded meaningful results. One randomized controlled trial (*n* = 96) of EMP+ for the treatment of BD began in 2008; its results are currently pending, according to the manufacturer's website ("Micronutrient-mood randomized controlled trials," 2008). If this and other well-designed trials provide evidence for the efficacy of multiple micronutrient supplements in treating BD, they may one day be helpful to pregnant women with BD. However, they would first have to be tested and found safe for use during pregnancy. The USDA warns women not to take dietary supplements or herbal products during pregnancy or breastfeeding without their doctors' approval and supervision, due to the harmful effects high doses of certain nutrients can have on babies ("Dietary Supplements", 2008). Vitamin A is one of the nutrients known to cause birth defects if taken in too high of a dose. It is one of the ingredients in EMP+. The United States government recommends pregnant women not take more than 10,000 IU of vitamin A daily ("Vitamin A in Your Pregnancy Diet", 2009). A typical initial daily dose of EMP+ (18 capsules) contains 6,912 IUs; dosage varies ("What Exactly is in Empowerplus?," 2003). Thus, if pregnant women ever considered taking EMP+ they would need to be certain that they did not exceed the upper limit of certain nutrients when added to their prenatal vitamin dosages and dietary intake.

Omega-3 fatty acids. Omega-3 fatty acids, otherwise referred to as fish oil, have received some empirical support for the treatment of BD. Results of a 4-month long, double-blind trial of 30 adults with BD who had had a manic or hypomanic episode within the year prior to the trial's start who were randomized to take either omega-3 fatty acids (9.6 grams daily) or an olive oil placebo in addition to treatment as usual indicated that those taking fish oil had a significantly longer period of remission than those taking placebos (Stoll et al., 1999). Post-treatment, they also had significantly improved ratings from baseline on all four of the outcome measures administered, which included the Young Mania Rating Scale (YMSR), Hamilton Rating Scale for Depression (HRSD),

Clinical Global Impression (CGI), and the Global Assessment Scale. The most common side effect in both the control and placebo group was mild gastrointestinal tract distress, most typically characterized by loose stools. Besides the small sample size, the fact that 86% of the treatment group participants were able to correctly guess which treatment group they belonged to (due to the capsules' reported "fishy aftertaste") was one of the only identified methodological flaws; therefore, a placebo effect could have influenced the results.

A larger, double-blind trial ($n = 75$) that supported the use of ethyl-eicosapentaenoic acid (ethyl-EPA, a type of omega-3 fatty acid) as an adjunctive treatment for depression in nonpregnant adults diagnosed with bipolar I or II disorder was conducted by Frangou, Lewis, and McCrone (2006). Individuals determined to be at risk of imminent suicide or hospitalization were excluded from the study. Subjects were randomly assigned to receive either 1gram daily of ethyl-EPA, 2 grams daily of ethyl-EPA, or a paraffin wax placebo for 12 weeks. Outcome measures included the HRSD, the YMSR, and the CGI. Results showed that those receiving ethyl-EPA had significantly improved HRSD and CGI scores when compared to the placebo group. The higher dosage of ethyl-EPA was just as effective as the lower dose. Mania scores did not differ between the placebo and control groups. The most commonly reported side effect by all three groups was loose stools (reported by 3 people in the placebo group, 3 people in the 1g ethyl-EPA daily group, and 6 people in the 2g ethyl-EPA daily group.)

This study provided evidence that ethyl-EPA may be an effective adjunctive treatment for nonsevere bipolar depression. It remains to be seen whether or not this finding will be replicated in pregnant women with BD. If it is, it seems likely that it would be safe for pregnant women with BD to take it as a dietary supplement, as fish oil is currently being recommended to the general population of pregnant women. The Mayo Clinic's website states the following:

Standard prenatal vitamins don't include omega-3 fatty acids, which help promote a baby's brain development. If you're unable or choose not to eat fish or other foods high in omega-3 fatty acids, your health care provider may recommend omega-3 fatty acid supplements in addition to prenatal vitamins. ("Prenatal Vitamins, Why They Matter, How to Choose," 2012, para. 6)

However, one researcher recommends that women with BD who take fish oil carefully watch for the development of any new mood symptoms, because there has been at least one reported case of a woman originally diagnosed with unipolar depression developing hypomanic symptoms five days after adding a supplement which contained two types of omega-3 fatty acids: docosahexanoic acid (DHA) and EPA (Kinrys, 2000). The woman was taking 1980 mg of DHA and 1320 mg of EPA daily.

St. John's wort. St. John's wort is the plant species *Hypericum perforatum*, also referred to as Klamath weed. It is used to treat mild depression; it was found to result in similar rates of major malformations in offspring born to 54 mothers exposed to St. John's wort during pregnancy as compared to 54 mothers exposed to antidepressants and 54 healthy mothers exposed to no teratogenic substances during pregnancy (Moretti, Maxson, Hanna, and Koren as cited in Dugoua, 2010). However, there is some evidence that it takes up to 6 weeks to become effective and may be associated with a switch to manic symptoms (Herbert-Ashton as cited in Harris, 2012; Nierenberg, Burt, Matthews, & Weiss, 1999). It appears that St. John's wort could possibly be helpful to some women with BD during pregnancy; however, given the minimal evidence of its safety and potentially serious side effects, it needs to be further studied before it can be recommended with confidence.

Exercise. The American College of Obstetricians and Gynecologists (2011) recommends that pregnant women exercise for "at least 30 minutes on most, if not all, days of the week" (para. 1). They also recommend that women start slowly and avoid exercises that require them to lie on their backs after the first trimester, as these exercises reduce blood flow to the womb. Da Costa, Rippen, Dritsa and Ring (2003) conducted a study on self-reported leisure-time physical activity during pregnancy and its relationship to psychological wellbeing. One-hundred eighty women currently in their first trimester of pregnancy participated. Inclusion criteria included being from 19 to 40 years old, married or in a stable relationship at the time of recruitment, and to have conceived naturally. Participants were interviewed about the frequency and duration of their physical activity during leisure time (not related to work) each trimester. Beginning in the third month of pregnancy, participants completed validated measures, which assessed for depression, anxiety, pregnancy-specific stressors, and fluctuations in daily stress level due to minor stressors, monthly. These measures included the Lubin depression adjective checklist Form C (DACL), the Pregnancy Experiences Questionnaire (PEQ), the state-trait anxiety inventory (STAI), and the Hassles Scale (revised). Results of the study showed that those who exercised in the first trimester had significantly lower rates of depression than those who did not exercise (15.1% versus 33.1%, respectively). Results were similar in the second trimester (5.7% of exercisers could be classified as depressed versus 18.9% of nonexercisers.) There were no group differences in rates of depression during the third trimester among exercisers and nonexercisers. Exercisers had lower state anxiety levels and pregnancy-specific stress scores than nonexercisers during each trimester. Exercisers reported statistically significant lower daily stress levels than nonexercisers during the first trimester of pregnancy. Differences in daily stress levels between the two groups did not reach statistical significance during the second and third trimesters.

Da Costa et al. (2003) concluded that low-intensity exercise is associated with reduced stress levels, anxiety, and depression during pregnancy. This conclusion seems to be supported by the data; however, the study had several limitations. Self-report was used to assess participants' levels of depression, anxiety, and stress, as well as their physical activity levels. It is possible that participants may have under- or over-reported any of these variables. It is also not clear whether exercise reduced participants' levels of depression, anxiety, and stress, or whether those who were already less anxious, depressed, and stressed engaged in more exercise. The results of this study suggest that the antidepressant effects of exercise, which have been evidenced in many randomized, controlled trials, may be extended to pregnant populations (Da Costa et al., 2003).

Although Da Costa et al. (2003) did not examine pregnant women with bipolar disorder specifically, their findings provide some support for the idea that exercise can be used to reduce stress, anxiety, and depression in pregnant women. Perhaps exercise could help pregnant women who experience bipolar depression improve their moods as well. As stress can trigger affective episodes, the stress relief provided by exercise could possibly help pregnant women with BD reduce their risk of experiencing new mood episodes. Further research on this topic should be conducted. It is not known whether or not mania can be triggered by exercise, however, a preliminary study of eight men and women with BD showed that most of them experienced a slight increase in manic symptoms for the first 2 weeks after beginning an exercise program, although their symptoms returned to base level after 2 weeks (Edenfield, 2008). Thus, pregnant women with BD who begin an exercise regimen should watch for early warning signs of mania or hypomania.

A controlled trial of the effectiveness of an exercise support program to treat postpartum depression was conducted in Taiwan (Heh, et al., 2008). Inclusion criteria included being married, aged 20-35 years old, having had no prior pregnancies, no history of psychiatric illness, and no obstetric complications. Sixty-three women who gave birth 4 weeks before the trial and had Edinburgh Postnatal Depression Scale (EPDS) scores above 10 at the time of recruitment finished the study. Participants were alternately assigned to an exercise intervention group or a control group. The exercise group members participated in an exercise program, which consisted of 3 hours of gentle stretching exercises weekly for 3 months; one hour of exercises were conducted in a hospital setting with five other participants, and group members were asked to do 2 or more hours at home. The investigator telephoned the experimental group participants weekly and reminded them to do the exercises. Members of the control group received standard care. All participants were asked to record their physical activity in 3-month records that they were given. The EPDS was administered 5 months after the trial's beginning.

Results indicated that after 5 months, 60.6% of the exercisers had EPDS scores below 10 versus 33.3% of the control group. The authors concluded that an exercise support program implemented during the postpartum period may contribute to psychological wellbeing. The authors' conclusions appear to be supported by the data. A larger sample size would have made the study's design stronger. Although women with prior psychiatric illnesses were excluded from this study, it is possible that postpartum women experiencing bipolar depression may experience the same mood benefits from initiating an exercise regimen. As mentioned previously, it would be prudent for pregnant women with BD who initiate an exercise routine to watch for any new mood symptoms that might develop in response to exercise, especially manic or hypomanic symptoms.

Yoga, mindfulness, and meditation. Shapiro et al. (2007) studied the effects of yoga as an adjunct to antidepressant medication for the treatment of people with unipolar depression who were in partial remission. Seventeen men and women attended six or more yoga sessions and completed both intake and post-intervention assessments. The yoga intervention they took part in consisted of 8 weeks of thrice-weekly, 60-90 minute sessions of Iyengar yoga. This method of yoga incorporates props, thereby allowing beginners to learn poses accurately and gradually, despite limited flexibility. It is taught by instructors who have undergone 3 years of rigorous training and have had their teaching skills certified by panels of senior teachers. Change in the HAM-D scores from intake to post-intervention was used as the main outcome measure of therapeutic effect. Participants' average pretreatment HAM-D score was 12.4. After the intervention, participants' average HAMD-D score was 6.2. Fifteen of the 17 completers showed a decrease in HAM-D scores.

The authors concluded that these results provide further evidence that yoga may be an effective complementary treatment for depression. This conclusion is based on weak data, as the trial lacked a control group and had a low number of participants who completed the study. Those participants included in the "completers" group only had to have attended 6 of the 20 yoga sessions offered; this added variability may have affected the study's results. Additionally, it is possible that regular participation in a social group was fully or partially responsible for the effects on depression. If yoga is, in fact, helpful in treating unipolar depression, it might be useful for the treatment of bipolar depression as well. It is possible that it could help to reduce the stress and depression levels of women with BD who are pregnant, too, although no studies of this topic have been published to date.

One preliminary study of mindfulness-based yoga's effects on maternal physical and psychological distress during pregnancy exists (Beddoe et al., 2009). Participants were 16 healthy women in their second and third trimesters of pregnancy. Inclusion criteria were as follows: at least 18 years old, first pregnancy, pregnant with only one child, and planning a hospital birth. Participants were excluded if they reported current psychiatric illness; used medications for depression, anxiety, sleep, or pain; had diabetes, hypertension, HIV or history of back surgery; or worked a nightshift. Participants underwent 7 weeks of Iyengar yoga combined with mindfulness-based stress reduction (MBSR). Beddoe et al. (2009) describe mindfulness as follows:

> A purposive process of learning how to pay attention from moment-to-moment to one's present experience while noticing and learning to let go of judgments and reactivity . . . In weekly sessions, mindfulness meditation skills were taught to help participants discover relationships between mindful practice and ability to

cope more effectively with stress using the following techniques: (a) body scan, a progressive relaxation in which participants direct attention and observe sensations; (b) sitting meditation, involving observation of one's breathing sensations, emotions, sound, and thoughts; (c) postural yoga, involving gentle physical poses integrated with breathing to develop strength, flexibility, and balance, no more strenuous than a 30 minute walk on flat ground; and (d) walking meditation, involving slow and observant walking. (p. 313)

The Perceived Stress Scale, the stressor subscale of the Prenatal Psychosocial Profile (PPP), and the State-Trait Anxiety Inventory (STAI) were used to assess participants' perceived stress and anxiety.

Significant reductions in perceived stress and trait anxiety resulted for women in their third trimester who initiated mindfulness-based yoga. Their pregnancy-specific stress and state anxiety scores stayed relatively stable. No significant changes in any of the four variables resulted for the eight women in their second trimester. The authors concluded that initiating a mindfulness-based yoga program during pregnancy is feasible and potentially efficacious in improving protective factors during pregnancy. Due to the small sample size and lack of a control group, these conclusions are tenuous. There is some preliminary evidence that a mindfulness-based cognitive therapy approach may be helpful in reducing affective symptoms of people with BD (Miklowitz et al., 2009). Beddoe et al.'s (2009) study did not delineate whether mindfulness or yoga would have produced the same effects if initiated independently. Professional organizations have not provided recommendations on the safety of yoga during pregnancy. Two of the study's initial participants dropped out, one due to preterm birth after the second yoga class and another due to preterm labor but not preterm birth after the third yoga class. It is impossible to know whether these pregnancy complications were directly related to yoga. Nonetheless, this study was useful because it suggested that pregnant women's levels of psychological distress could potentially be reduced via mindfulness-based yoga. If this is supported by randomized, controlled trials in the future, and if the safety of yoga is established for the pregnant population, perhaps mindfulness-based yoga may also prove to be helpful in relieving psychological distress of pregnant women with BD. At the moment, however, this intervention seems to lack the amount of evidence that would justify recommending it to pregnant women with BD.

Chapter III

Methods

Research Design

The purpose of this study was to identify key concerns and needs of women with BD related to pregnancy and the postpartum period. The women included those who were anticipating becoming pregnant in the future, those who were currently pregnant, and those who had children. The research was conducted using an online survey and by telephone interviews of women with BD. The main areas of inquiry in the study were (a) key concerns and perceived challenges regarding BD and pregnancy, (b) perceptions of partner support, (c) psychosocial coping strategies and use of complementary medicine, (c) perceptions of appropriate medication use, (e) information sources utilized, and (f) recommendations women with BD would give to others contemplating pregnancy.

Participants

Participants were 38 women over the age of 18 who indicated that they had BD and that they had received a diagnosis of BD (type I or II) by a psychiatrist. Online survey participants ($n = 31$) were women who responded to a posting and online link posted on Craigslist volunteer boards in major cities across the United States. Telephone survey participants ($n = 7$) were recruited via messages sent to a Facebook group for women with BD who were pregnant or had previously given birth.

In total, 97 individuals accessed the online questionnaire and 31 individuals provided data. Of those who did not provide data, 19 entered no information and 47 provided demographic data but did not respond to any survey questions. Of the 31 participants, 77% responded to all of the questions presented ($n = 24$) and the remainder of participants answered most but not all of the questions ($n = 7$).

Measures

Three versions of an open-ended survey were used to inquire about online and telephone participants' attitudes and experiences regarding pregnancy. The three versions of the survey were tailored to the three groups of participants: (a) women who had never given birth (see Appendix H), (b) women who were pregnant at the time of survey administration (see Appendix I), and (c) women who had previously given birth (see Appendix J).

Procedures

The following study procedures were approved by the Institutional Review Board of Alliant International University. Telephone surveys were used to interview participants because they allowed me to ask follow-up, probing questions in response to participants' answers to the survey questions. This allowed me to clarify their responses and obtain greater detail. Online questionnaires were used because they were thought to be a more convenient, more confidential method for some women to participate. Given the amount of stigma surrounding mental illness in our society, it was presumed that some women with BD would be more comfortable participating in this survey in the more removed fashion that the Internet allows.

The online survey was created using Qualtrics software. A link to the questionnaire was posted on Craigslist volunteer boards in major cities across the United States (see Appendix A). When potential participants accessed the link they were led to several pages informing them of the study, the inclusion requirements, and time involved in participation (see Appendix B); the rights and risks of participation including assurances of confidentiality via consent form (see Appendix C); and a third page where participants were given the option to be interviewed via telephone or complete the online survey (see Appendix D). Telephone survey participants were also recruited via messages sent to a Facebook group for women with BD who were pregnant or had previously given birth. These potential interview participants were asked to email the author should they wish to participate and then electronically sign and return an Informed Consent Form via email before arranging a telephone appointment. In the form, they were given space to select available times for the interview (see Appendix E). They were called at their selected available times and asked questions to confirm their eligibility to participate (see Appendix F). Those who completed online surveys were directed to a similar, brief demographic form (see Appendix G). Both telephone and on-line participants were given the same surveys. For all participants, the surveys administered were specific to the following three conditions: those who were not pregnant and had never given birth (see Appendix H), those who were currently pregnant (see Appendix I), and those who had previously given birth (see Appendix J). Telephone interviews were more semi-structured in that follow up questions were asked. Participants received no financial incentive for participation.

Data Analysis

The data of this study consisted of open-ended responses to online survey questions and transcripts from telephone interviews. Qualitative research is focused on uncovering knowledge about the way participants think and feel regarding the issues presented by the researcher. This qualitative analysis utilized an inductive reasoning approach, in which patterns in the data were identified via thematic codes, in order to interpret and structure the meaning derived from the data. Patton (1980) noted, "Inductive analysis means that the patterns, themes, and categories of analysis come from the data; they emerge out of the data rather than being imposed on them prior to data collection and analysis" (p. 306).

I transcribed telephone interviews and reviewed Qualtrics online survey responses. Following this, I worked with my dissertation chair, a psychology professor. We independently read the transcripts and questionnaire responses and identified key themes by using the constant comparative method, wherein segments of the transcripts and questionnaires are reviewed and codes are assigned that fit the concepts implied by the data (Strauss & Corbin, 1990). Emblematic quotations were highlighted and we agreed on a set of key themes. By using this method, I documented various aspects of BD and pregnancy that were important to the participants. The transcripts and other content collected from the participants were examined several times in order to sort responses into the identified themes.

Chapter IV

Results

Introduction

The purpose of this study was to explore the concerns women with BD may have regarding pregnancy issues. Although there has been a great deal of recent research about the treatment of BD during pregnancy that is aimed at healthcare providers, little information is available on the comprehensive and holistic management of BD during pregnancy that is directed towards women with BD. This chapter presents the responses of the 38 women with BD who participated in this study by completing online questionnaires or telephone surveys. This chapter begins with a description of the participant sample, comments on the validity of the questionnaires and interviews, and presents key themes that emerged from analysis of the interviews. Representative quotes that best demonstrate the content of each theme are provided.

Participant Characteristics

Of the 38 participants, 31 completed the online questionnaire and 7 chose to participate in the telephone interview. All participants reported that they had received a diagnosis of BD from a psychiatrist, either BD-I ($n = 20$) or BD-II ($n = 18$). The age of the participants varied from 19 to 62 years of age ($M = 32.34$, $SD = 11.42$). Seventy-nine percent of the participants self-identified as Caucasian or "White" ($n = 30$). The remainder of participants self-identified as Asian (8%, $n = 3$), African American (3%, $n = 1$), Latina (3%, $n = 1$), or of mixed race (8%, $n = 3$). Participants included women who had previously given birth ($n = 21$), women who were not pregnant and had never given birth ($n = 14$), and women who were currently pregnant and had never given birth ($n = 3$).

One of the women who had previously given birth was 21 weeks pregnant. The three participants who were pregnant and had never given birth were from 13 to 24 weeks pregnant ($M = 19.67$, $SD = 5.86$). The participants who had previously given birth had between 1 and 5 children ($M = 2.19$, $SD = 1.08$) whose ages ranged from 0.8 to 39 years ($M = 14.75$, $SD = 11.52$).

Validity of the Interviews

The participants who were interviewed via telephone appeared to be engaged in the interview; they provided detailed and lengthy responses to the open-ended questions which were also posed by the online questionnaire. Although they were not told that the interview had any particular required duration, they remained on the phone between 30 and 90 minutes. Several of the participants thanked me after the experience, indicating that they wished that more information were available regarding BD and pregnancy. Several participants expressed a willingness to continue the survey in the future should I have follow-up questions. All interview participants asked for a summary of the survey results upon completion of the project.

Many of the online survey participants provided detailed answers to the questions; whereas others gave shorter answers. All 31 participants provided useful material that could be interpreted for this study. Time spent completing the online surveys varied from approximately 8 to 71 minutes ($M = 23.6$, $SD = 16.68$). Fifty-eight percent ($n = 18$) of the online survey participants provided their email addresses and asked that I send them a summary of the survey findings once my research was complete.

Key Themes

Online and phone interview results have been integrated in this section. The results of the survey questions that addressed similar topics have been combined to

reduce redundancy. Key themes described in this section are presented in Table 1. The

most commonly reported themes and subthemes are elaborated upon in greater detail in

the narrative portion of this section, and the tables present an exhaustive account of the

varied responses.

Table 1

Key Themes

Chief concerns, fears, and information desired regarding BD and pregnancy

Experiences of mood episodes during pregnancy and postpartum

Experiences and plans regarding pregnancy medication regimens

Partner's preparedness and information needed to be supportive regarding BD and
pregnancy

Sources used and recommended to gain information about BD and pregnancy

Information participants wish they had known and advice they would give to others

Coping with challenging aspects of pregnancy or considering becoming pregnant

Stress reduction and complementary medicine methods participants tried or would
consider trying to help manage BD during pregnancy

Other information participants would like included in an informational resource about
BD and pregnancy

Chief concerns, fears, and information desired regarding BD and pregnancy.

Table 2a and 2b present participants' chief concerns, fears, and information desired

regarding the ways BD affects pregnancy and the postpartum period. Participants who

were currently pregnant or had previously given birth were asked to recall the concerns

they had prior to becoming pregnant or describe the fears and concerns they would have

should they consider having another child. Participants' responses fell under four key themes: fear of re-emergent mental illness, concerns about BD treatment, parenting concerns, and interpersonal/relationship concerns.

Fear of re-emergent mental illness. Of the entire sample, 87% described fears of re-emergent BD symptoms during pregnancy and the postpartum period. The most common re-emergent mental illness fears were that of experiencing intensified symptoms of BD symptoms, mood swings, or having a relapse of BD during pregnancy. For example, one participant (#32) stated, "I'm worried about mood swings, because when I was first pregnant, I had really, really bad depression, hypomania, and rage episodes. And I couldn't control the emotions." The second most common re-emergent illness fears were of postpartum depression or postpartum psychosis.

Five participants who had previously given birth reported that they experienced urges to complete suicide or inflict self-harm during pregnancy or the postpartum stage. Five participants who had never given birth and were not currently pregnant expressed fears that they, too, would consider suicide or self-harm should they become pregnant. Three participants who had never given birth and were not pregnant expressed concerns about the teratogenic effects of mood episodes experienced during pregnancy.

Concerns about BD treatment. Of the entire sample, 76% described concerns about how to treat BD during pregnancy and the postpartum period. The most common treatment concern was stopping or changing medication (reported by 14 participants who had previously given birth and 11 participants who had not previously given birth and were not currently pregnant). For example, one participant (#37) stated, "I would end up in a mental hospital for the whole 9 months, no doubt, if I went off my medications, so that's obviously a big fear."

Table 2a

Chief Concerns, Fears, and Information Desired regarding BD and Pregnancy- I

Theme/Subtheme	Number of Participants who Reported Theme		
	Pre-Pregnancy ($n = 14$)	Currently Pregnant ($n = 3$)	Post-Pregnancy ($n = 21$)
Fear of Re-emergent Mental Illness	14 (100%)	2 (67%)	17 (81%)
Worse symptoms/mood swings/relapse during pregnancy	10	1	12
Postpartum depression/postpartum psychosis	8	2	10
Pregnancy hormones' effect on mood	6	1	4
Losing control/losing sanity/hospitalization	5	0	5
Suicide/self-harm	5	0	5
Teratogenic effects of mood episodes	3	0	0
Excessive weight gain due to impulsive eating when depressed	1	0	1
Losing my job due to BD episodes during pregnancy	1	0	0
Deciding whether or not to have an abortion should BD symptoms become unmanageable	0	0	1
Concerns about BD Treatment	13 (92%)	0 (0%)	16 (76%)
Stopping or changing medication	11	0	14
Teratogenic effects of taking medication while pregnant	9	0	9
Teratogenic effects of taking medication while nursing	1	0	4
Healthcare providers' perceived lack of knowledge/ misinformed statements	1	0	4
Finding complementary methods to treat BD	2	0	3
Finding a psychotherapist/support networks/resources	2	0	1
How to prepare for pregnancy with BD	1	0	2
No longer able to self-medicate BD symptoms with alcohol/drugs due to pregnancy	1	0	1
Post-delivery psychiatric care	0	0	1

Table 2b

Chief Concerns, Fears, and Information Desired regarding BD and Pregnancy- II

Theme/Subtheme	Number of Participants who Reported Theme		
	Pre-Pregnancy ($n = 14$)	Currently Pregnant ($n = 3$)	Post-Pregnancy ($n = 21$)
Parenting Concerns	8 (57%)	1 (33%)	11 (52%)
Genetic risks of children developing BD	6	0	7
Deciding whether or not to have children	3	0	3
Fear of BD negatively affecting parenting skills	3	0	2
Fear of harming children or baby	2	0	3
Fear of being unable to bond with baby due to BD	2	0	2
Grief/frustration over lost joyous pregnancy and childbirth	1	1	1
Interpersonal/Relationship Concerns	6 (43%)	1 (33%)	6 (29%)
Dealing with stigma/guilt/judgments of self and others	4	0	4
Fear of damaging relationship with partner	2	1	2
Fear of destroying relationships in general	3	0	0
Other	7 (50%)	1 (33%)	14 (67%)
Was not diagnosed with BD prior to pregnancy	0	0	7
Did not seek information about BD and pregnancy	1	1	3
Did not know what to be concerned about	2	0	2
Wanted to hear about other women's experiences	2	0	2
Was not worried about BD and pregnancy	0	1	1
Pregnancy was unplanned	0	0	2
Wanted to hear positive information and experiences about BD and pregnancy	0	0	1
Wanted to know how to put a child genetically predisposed to BD up for adoption	1	0	0
Was over 35 years old when pregnant	0	0	1
Experienced infertility	1	0	0

The second most common treatment concern was the teratogenic effects of psychotropic medications used during and prior to pregnancy. Participants expressed a desire to know the various BD medications' rates of fetal abnormalities and longer-term developmental deficits that could occur in children exposed to them in utero. Several participants expressed concern about the lack of research available regarding the consequences of taking medications during pregnancy. For example, one participant (#33) expressed a desire to know, "How 'safe' are the medications approved for use during pregnancy? What types of birth defects do they produce and at what rate? Would my psychiatrist take them if she were in my shoes?" Several participants expressed a belief that it is never acceptable to use psychotropic medications while pregnant.

Five participants expressed a desire to find appropriate complementary medicine methods to help manage BD symptoms during pregnancy, and some of them wondered whether or not they would be candidates for using complementary medicine instead of traditional psychotropic medications. Five participants expressed concerns that their healthcare providers may not have the knowledge and expertise required to help them to most effectively manage their high-risk pregnancies. A 30-year old participant with three children (#27) stated, "I was told by a nurse that women with BD shouldn't become mothers because they could physically and/or mentally abuse their children."

Parenting concerns. Of the entire sample, 53% described concerns and fears regarding the ways that BD may negatively affect parenting. The most common parenting concern was about the genetic risk of one's child developing BD. Participants who mentioned this concern wanted to know the probability of their child developing BD. They also wanted to know if there were any ways to reduce the likelihood of their child developing BD, and which early warning signs of the illness they should look for in their children so that they could implement treatment as soon as possible.

The second most common concern was deciding whether or not to have children. This theme was related to an ethical dilemma and guilt about giving birth to a child who may suffer as participants had from the pain that BD causes. The decision was also linked to some participants' concern that BD could negatively affect their parenting skills. For example, one 27-year old participant (#37) without children who was in the process of acquiring a tubal ligation to prevent pregnancy expressed her concerns as follows:

> If I had a kid with BD, I'd feel that every time they were in pain, I'd be in pain, because I'm the one that gave it to them . . . And sometimes I find it hard to take care of myself, and so to be responsible for another life is something I don't think would be responsible for me to do . . . I believe that to be a good mom, I would need to be consistent, and I'm not consistent with anything.

She also expressed concern that her antipsychotic medication had such a strong sedative effect that she would sleep through her baby's crying.

Five participants reported the fear that they might harm their unborn babies or their older children during pregnancy or the postpartum period due to uncontrolled BD mood symptoms. For example, one participant (#36) said:

> You hear lots of scary things about moms committing suicide or hurting their babies. I never had any of those symptoms or wanted to hurt my baby. If anything, after the hospital, I was disinterested in my baby, because I was drugged up and out of it. But I worry if it happened again, the symptoms may be different.

Four participants worried that their ability to bond with their newborn babies would be hindered by postpartum mood episodes. Three participants reported fears of missing out on the joyous post-delivery time they imagined they would experience if they did not have BD. For example, one participant (#25) disclosed:

> I'm concerned about how I will hold up after the due date. It's supposed to be such a joyous, happy moment when bringing a life into the world. I'm afraid my

moods will make me see otherwise, and that would be horrible.

Interpersonal/relationship concerns. Of the entire sample, 34% reported concerns about interpersonal issues. The most commonly experienced interpersonal issue was feeling judged and stigmatized regarding the decision to become pregnant given their BD diagnosis. One participant (#33) reported, "My mother has told me that I shouldn't get pregnant. That really hurt." The second most commonly reported interpersonal theme was fear that becoming pregnant would damage their relationships with their romantic partner.

Experiences of mood episodes during pregnancy and postpartum. Table 3 presents participants' experiences of mood episodes during pregnancy and the postpartum period, as well as the factors they attribute to the development of these mood episodes or lack of mood episodes. This question was only posed to women who were currently pregnant or who had previously given birth, as it did not apply to those who had not previously experienced pregnancy.

Participants who experienced a mood episode during pregnancy or postpartum. Fourteen participants reported experiencing a mood episode during pregnancy or the postpartum period. The majority of these participants reported experiencing a depressive episode ($n = 8$), and half of them reported that they also became suicidal ($n = 4$). Most participants attributed the mood episodes they experienced during pregnancy and the postpartum period to hormonal changes associated with pregnancy, stress, and foregoing medication. For example, one participant (#12) reported, "I had many mood episodes. I was feeling very suicidal and worthless. I really was a complete basket case. I attributed them to the raging hormones and not being medicated."

Table 3

Experiences of Mood Episodes During Pregnancy and Postpartum

Themes/Sub-themes	Number of Participants who Reported Theme	
	Currently Pregnant ($n = 3$)	Post-Pregnancy ($n = 21$)
Participant experienced a mood episode during pregnancy or postpartum	2	13
Participant experienced a depressive episode	1	7
Participant became suicidal	0	4
Participant experienced a mixed episode	1	2
Participant experienced a manic episode	1	1
Causes attributed to the mood episodes participants experienced during pregnancy		
Hormonal changes associated with pregnancy	2	4
Stress	2	3
Foregoing psychotropic medication/ineffective medication	0	4
Romantic partner relationship difficulties	0	2
Lack of self-nurturing	0	1
Poor body image associated with being pregnant	0	1
Somatic concerns (lack of sleep, pain associated with pregnancy)	0	1
Not being diagnosed with BD prior to pregnancy	0	1
Participant did not experience a mood episode during pregnancy	0	7
Mood was better than usual/more stable while pregnant	0	4
Causes attributed to the lack of mood episodes during pregnancy		
Thrilled to have another child	0	2
Strong support system	0	1
Educated regarding BD and pregnancy/knew what to expect	0	1
Medication	0	1
Unsure about cause	0	1
Other		
Some BD symptoms improved but some were worse	0	1

Participants who did not experience a mood episode during pregnancy or postpartum. Seven participants who had previously given birth reported that they did not experience any mood episodes during pregnancy or the postpartum period. Four of these participants stated that their mood improved and that they felt more stable during pregnancy than they had felt prior to pregnancy. For example, one participant (#31) who had given birth to two children and was 21 weeks pregnant at the time she participated in the survey stated, "My mood has been fantastic this pregnancy and I think this is because I have known to expect severe episodes and have had support on hand in case this happened." Another participant (#38) said, "I had no mood episodes during pregnancy, probably due to the medication and having a good outlook; I was happy and content to be pregnant, even when I got gestational diabetes and my health changed and I had to give myself shots."

Experiences and plans regarding pregnancy medication regimens. Table 4 presents participants' experiences with medication use during pregnancy and their decisions regarding how to change medication regimens. Participants who had never been pregnant reported their plans about medication use.

Experiences and plans regarding medication use during pregnancy. Of the entire sample, 34% reported that they forewent medication use during pregnancy or they were planning to forego medication out of concern for teratogenic effects (reported by seven participants who had previously given birth, four participants who had not previously given birth and were not currently pregnant, and two participants who had not previously given birth and were currently pregnant). One participant (#33) stated, "What's best for the baby is whole foods and natural everything; that's what our bodies are meant to do- have kids- not have a bunch of foreign substances in them." Six participants who had previously been pregnant or who were currently pregnant indicated that they had planned to forego medication use, but either the manifestation of a new mood episode or the fear of one made them resume using medication mid-way through their pregnancies. For example, one participant (#2) reported, "I was not on medication when I became pregnant. I stayed that way until I was hospitalized at 15.5 weeks, and they decided there was more risk to the baby with me being unmedicated than the risk of medication."

Experiences and plans regarding determining how to alter medication regimen. Of the entire sample, 45% indicated that they determined whether or not to change their medication regimen or that they would make this decision in the future by consulting with medical professionals, including psychiatrists, OB/GYNs, doctors, nurses, and/or pharmacists. Some participants indicated that getting a second opinion before making medication changes was or would be important to them. One participant (#28) said, "I will discontinue taking all medications while pregnant regardless of doctor recommendations or pregnancy risk levels. I don't want any psychiatric medications affecting my baby's development."

Table 4

Experiences and Plans Regarding Pregnancy Medication Regimen

Theme/Subtheme	Number of Participants who Reported Theme		
	Pre-Pregnancy ($n = 14$)	Currently Pregnant ($n = 3$)	Post-Pregnancy ($n = 21$)
Experiences and plans regarding medication use during pregnancy			
Stopped or will stop using all medication before becoming pregnant in order to prevent teratogenic effects	4	2	7
Did not use medication during the beginning of pregnancy but resumed medication use later during the pregnancy (due to a mood episode or to prevent one from occurring)	0	2	4
Used or will use only medications which pose no risk of teratogenic effects	3	0	2
Used or will use medication during entire pregnancy	1	0	4
Experienced much trial and error to determine effective medication regimen during pregnancy that caused minimal side effects	0	1	3
Tried or will try psychotherapy or complementary treatments (ECT, TMS, herbal medicine, vitamins) to manage BD during pregnancy	2	0	2
Experiences and plans regarding determining how to alter medication regimen			
Spoke with or will speak with psychiatrist/doctor/ARNP/pharmacist/OB/GYN	6	2	9
Obtained or will obtain a second opinion	3	0	1
Educated or will educate myself about BD and pregnancy	2	0	1
Healthcare providers disagreed with each other regarding the best medication regimen for participant	0	1	1
Healthcare provider and participant disagreed about the best medication regimen for participant	0	1	0
Unsure of how to make medication decisions regarding BD and pregnancy	1	0	0
Did not alter medication regimen or consult about it during pregnancy	0	0	1
Was not diagnosed with BD prior to pregnancy	0	0	1

Partner's preparedness and information needed to be supportive regarding BD and pregnancy. Tables 5a and 5b present information about participants' romantic partners' preparedness to be supportive to them during pregnancy with regards to BD. Participants who had not previously been pregnant were asked to respond to questions regarding how they imagined they would help their partners to be supportive to them during pregnancy and the postpartum periods. Participants' responses fell into two key themes; these pertained to information participants felt would be necessary for their partners to know in order to be supportive to them during pregnancy, and the sources of this information that they utilized. Twelve participants indicated that their partners had not been prepared to support them during pregnancy regarding issues related to BD. Five participants who had previously given birth indicated that their partners had been prepared to support them this way.

Information and resources partner needed or will need in order to be supportive. Of the entire sample, 29% (5 participants who had previously given birth, 1 participant who had not previously given birth and was not currently pregnant, and 5 participants who had not previously given birth and were currently pregnant) indicated that they believed one's partner must be aware of the risks associated with BD and pregnancy and have a sense of what to expect during and after pregnancy in order to be an effective support person. Six participants stated they thought it would be important for their partners to identify and recognize symptoms of BD they typically exhibited when experiencing a relapse. For example, one participant (#29) stated, "If my partner has never seen me "unmedicated," as I *hate* to say, they will obviously not fully understand. My partner would need to know the realities of my disease and which symptoms of the disease affect me, personally."

How partner obtained information needed in order to be supportive. Of the

entire sample, 43% indicated that their romantic partners had accompanied or would

accompany them to their doctor, psychiatrist, and psychologist appointments in order to

learn how BD may influence pregnancy and the postpartum period, as well as learn how

to best support participants. Participants seemed to view their partner attending

appointments as supportive acts in and of themselves, not just as a means of gaining

information. For example, one participant (#36) who was diagnosed with BD after

suffering from postpartum psychosis described that gratitude that she felt by being

accompanied to her appointments as follows:

> [At] the follow-up appointments with the psychiatrist, I was kind of in disbelief. I
> wasn't even listening to the doctor sometimes. Having someone there to really
> listen and make sure you understand your treatment plan [was essential]. I would
> leave the doctor's office like, "So how many pills am I supposed to take?" and if I
> had been there by myself, I don't know how I would have gotten through it.

Table 5a

Partner's Preparedness and Information Needed to be Supportive regarding BD and Pregnancy- I

Theme/Subtheme	Number of Participants who Reported Theme		
	Pre-Pregnancy (*n* = 14)	Currently Pregnant (*n* = 3)	Post-Pregnancy (*n* = 21)
Partner was not prepared to be supportive during pregnancy	N/A	2	10
Partner was prepared to be supportive during pregnancy	N/A	0	5
Information and resources partner needed or will need in order to be supportive			
Risks of BD and pregnancy/what to expect during and after pregnancy	5	1	5
Symptoms of BD participant typically experiences	4	0	2
When to take participant to the doctor/hospital	2	0	1
How to comfort and listen to participant	1	0	2
How to care for their other children or hire childcare	0	0	3
How to self-soothe when participant becomes irritable	0	0	2
Risks of stopping medication use/reasons participant must continue to use medication	2	0	0
Ability to provide financial support	1	0	1
Genetic risks of BD in children	0	0	1
How partner did/would obtain information needed in order to be supportive			
Partner accompanied participant to doctor/psychiatrist/psychologist appointments	9	0	3
Participant provided partner with necessary information	1	1	5
Partner conducted Internet research	3	0	1
Couples' counseling	0	0	3
Partner read books or pamphlets (e.g., *Loving Someone with Bipolar Disorder*)	0	1	1
Partner participated in his or her own psychotherapy	0	0	1
Participant's parents provided partner with necessary information	0	0	1

Table 5b

Partner's Preparedness and Information Needed to be Supportive regarding BD and Pregnancy- II

Theme/Subtheme	Number of Participants who Reported Theme		
	Pre-Pregnancy (*n* = 14)	Currently Pregnant (*n* = 3)	Post-Pregnancy (*n* = 21)
Participants' Recommendations			
Be open and honest with partner	2	0	1
Have partner join support group with other partners who have dealt with this issue	1	0	1
Additional Reflections			
Partner was not supportive postpartum	0	0	1
Has not disclosed BD diagnosis to partner	1	0	0
Did not know how partner could become prepared to support participant	1	0	0

Sources used and recommended to gain information about BD and pregnancy. Tables 6a and 6b present the sources that participants used and would recommend that others use in order to learn about the ways BD may affect pregnancy and the postpartum period. Participants' responses fell into three key themes: *Conversations with healthcare providers, Websites,* and *Non-Internet resources.*

Conversations with healthcare providers. Of the entire sample, 76% participants reported speaking with or recommending that others speak with healthcare providers to gain information about BD and pregnancy. Conversations with psychiatrists were the most frequently recommended or used means of gaining information. Four participants indicated that they believed it was important for women with BD to work with psychiatrists who had expertise in treating pregnancy issues among women with BD. An important concern endorsed by several participants in response to several survey questions was that healthcare providers often lacked the knowledge or experience necessary to provide them with accurate information and adequate care. Noting her belief that some practitioners also prefer not to treat pregnant women with BD, one participant (#34) noted:

> My obstetrician didn't know anything about treating women with BD. And I went to a hospital and the medical staff there didn't know. You need someone who's really well-informed. They don't want to be liable, so they don't want to touch it.

Another participant (#23) echoed this concern and expressed feelings of frustration over her healthcare providers never providing her with "concrete" answers to her questions about BD and pregnancy.

The second most commonly reported type of healthcare provider participants spoke with or recommended speaking with were primary care physicians. Ten participants recommended that others speak with obstetricians, and five participants recommended they speak with psychologists, therapists, or social workers. A few participants reported that gaining information by speaking with naturopathic doctors, support groups, pharmacists, physicians who specialize in abortion, electroconvulsive therapy or transcranial magnetic stimulation providers, and/or nutritionists was or would be helpful.

Websites. Of the entire sample, 71% reported using or recommending that others use the Internet to gain information about BD and pregnancy. Fifteen participants used or recommended peer support websites about women's experiences, including blogs and message boards. Depression and Bipolar Support Alliance, Yahoo Answers, and HealthyPlace.com were specifically mentioned. One woman indicated that she did not recommend peer support websites because she found that the advice varied too much.

Twelve participants used or recommended looking at websites staffed by mental health

providers, including those of the National Alliance on Mental Illness, the National

Institute of Mental Health, The American Psychological Association, PubMED, 211.org,

babymed.com, and WebMD.

Non-Internet resources. Of the entire sample, 32% reported using or

recommending that others use non-Internet resources to gain information about BD and

pregnancy. Books or magazines were the most frequently recommended or used non-

Internet resources. One participant (#6) who had previously given birth stated that she

read Kristen Finn's book, *Bipolar and Pregnant: How to Manage and Succeed in

Planning and Parenting while Living with Manic Depression.* She commented that

although she was not satisfied with this book, "It's the only one out there" on the subject.

Table 6a

Sources Used and Recommended to Gain Information about BD and Pregnancy- I

Theme/Subtheme	Number of Participants who Reported Theme		
	Pre-Pregnancy ($n = 14$)	Currently Pregnant ($n = 3$)	Post-Pregnancy ($n = 21$)
Conversations with Healthcare Providers	12 (86%)	3 (100%)	14 (67%)
Psychiatrist	7	1	9
Primary care physician	7	2	5
OB/GYN	4	2	4
Psychologist/therapist/social worker	2	1	2
Recommended finding a psychiatrist or OB with expertise in treating pregnancy and BD	2	0	2
Support group	1	0	2
ECT & TMS specialists	1	0	0
Nutritionist	1	0	0
Naturopathic doctor	1	0	0
Pharmacist	1	0	0
Abortion physician	0	0	1
Recommended speaking openly and candidly with clinicians	0	1	0
Websites	11 (79%)	2 (67%)	14 (67%)
Peer support websites	8	0	7
Websites staffed by mental health providers	4	2	6
Unspecified Websites	3	0	4
Psychiatrist	7	1	9
Non-Internet Resources	2 (14%)	0 (0%)	7 (33%)
Books, magazines	2	0	7
Teratogenic medication lawsuit commercial	0	0	1
WIIC	0	0	1

Table 6b

Sources Used and Recommended to Gain Information about BD and Pregnancy- II

Theme/Subtheme	Number of Participants Who Reported Theme		
	Pre-Pregnancy ($n = 14$)	Currently Pregnant ($n = 3$)	Post-Pregnancy ($n = 21$)
Additional Reflections	0 (0%)	1 (33%)	10 (48%)
Did not know where to look for information	0	0	5
Did not look for information before pregnancy	0	1	2
Gained information from conversations with non-clinicians (partner, church leader)	0	0	2
Not diagnosed with BD prior to pregnancy	0	0	2
Information found made them feel scared and guilty	0	0	1

Information participants wish they had known in retrospect and advice they would give to others. The question pertaining to the information participants wished they had known in retrospect, as well as the advice they would give to others who were considering pregnancy, was only administered to women who were currently pregnant or who had previously given birth, as it did not apply to those who had not previously experienced pregnancy. Participants' responses fell under three key themes: *Information about preparing for pregnancy, Information about pregnancy,* and *Information about the postpartum period.*

Information about preparing for pregnancy. Of the entire sample, 67% reported wishing they had known more about pregnancy with BD or wanting to share advice with others regarding how to best prepare. An equal number of participants endorsed the top three subthemes, which were (a) become educated about BD and pregnancy issues prior to conception, (b) have a strong support network in place prior to pregnancy, and (c) carefully consider the decision of whether or not to have children. Five participants who had previously given birth and one participant who had not previously given birth and was currently pregnant stated that educating oneself about the risks of pregnancy and the postpartum period with BD and having a strong support system (i.e., a psychiatrist, therapist, OB, general physician, romantic partner) in place prior to becoming pregnant were important. For example, one participant (#2) shared:

> I wish I had known I needed to get care *right away* when I found out I was pregnant, instead of waiting until I was hospitalized at 15 weeks. Make sure you are *stable*, make sure you have a large and tight-knit support group, make sure you have a primary care, OB/midwife, a psychiatrist, and a counselor *before* you get pregnant . . . Be prepared to feel "crazier" than you ever have. Accept now that this will be difficult and fully commit as a family to making it through the pregnancy intact. That sounds so simple, but pregnancy mood swings on top of bipolar cycles (if you relapse) make that harder to do. Make sure that you can leave work and still pay the bills. There is a chance you will face that situation, maybe even pretty early in the pregnancy.

The other most frequently noted aspect of preparing for pregnancy that participants wished they had considered or wanted to share with others was to carefully consider the decision of whether or not to have children. Two women stated that they would advise a friend with BD not to have children, while two would advise them that BD should not necessarily stop a person from becoming pregnant. One participant (#38), a 43-year old mother of a 6-year old daughter stated:

> Nobody ever warned us about the reality and demands an infant makes on you as a person. I still have trouble structuring my day, and with an infant, you need to feed them and have them rest on a schedule. If you can't put that in place, it will make things harder. So you have to look at your own limitations and be brutally honest . . . But once the struggle of the whole thing was over, the ultimate joy of having a child is worth everything I've gone through [postpartum mania, suicide attempt, hospitalization and ECT] to have her here. And that's a universal feeling. Once a person has a child, it's like, "Holy cow!" and you would never *not* do it again.

Information about pregnancy. Of the entire sample, 58% reported wishing they had known more information about, or that they would like to share advice with others regarding, how to best manage BD while pregnant. The most common advice participants would share with others or wished they had known during pregnancy was to participate in psychotherapy during pregnancy. For example, one participant (#30) shared this advice: "Check in with a therapist regularly . . . doctors usually are too rushed."

The second most frequently reported advice participants (four participants who had previously given birth) would share with others or wished they had known during pregnancy was to *not* attempt to forego all psychotropic medication during pregnancy. For example, one participant (#4) stated, "Going on medication is never bad. My thought is that if you are going to kill yourself then medication will be the best. I thought I was going to totally lose it, and then I restarted my medication at 17 weeks and I never felt better."

Information about the postpartum period. Two participants mentioned advice or information they wished they had known about the postpartum period. One participant (#9) reported, "I wish I would have known that I would have severe PPD. I could have prepared myself mentally and emotionally and sought medication adjustment earlier." Table 7a and 7b present information participants wish they had known about the effects of BD on pregnancy and the postpartum period in retrospect, as well as the advice they would give to others who were considering becoming pregnant.

Table 7a

Information Participants Wish They Had Known & Advice They Would Give to Others- I

Themes/Subthemes	Number of Participants Who Reported Theme	
	Currently Pregnant ($n = 3$)	Post-Pregnancy ($n = 21$)
Information about Preparing for Pregnancy	1 (33%)	15 (71%)
Educate yourself about risks of pregnancy and postpartum with BD	1	5
Have a support system in place prior to pregnancy (including psychiatrist, therapist, OB, GP, and romantic partner)	1	5
Learn about genetic risks to child/do genetic counseling session	0	3
Make sure you're stable before becoming pregnant	1	2
Discuss medications (including teratogenic effects) thoroughly with your doctor	0	2
Consider parenting stress' effects on BD symptoms	0	2
Consider the decision to become pregnant carefully	0	2
Prevent unplanned pregnancy	0	2
Do not get pregnant	0	2
Do not let BD necessarily stop you from getting pregnant	0	2
Be financially prepared to leave work if needed	1	0
Information about Pregnancy	2 (67%)	12 (57%)
Participate in psychotherapy	1	4
Don't try to forego medication during entire pregnancy	0	4
Take medication which is safe for the fetus or decrease medication	0	3
Seek medical care as soon as you know you are pregnant	1	2
Join a support group and attend regularly	0	2
Try complementary medicine (light therapy, herbal/nutrition therapy, or acupuncture)	0	2
Recognize early symptoms and learn how to intervene with them	0	1
Talk to your psychiatrist often	0	1
Don't be ashamed to ask for help	0	1
Exercise	0	1
Consider abortion as a possible option	0	1

Table 7b

Information Participants Wish They Had Known & Advice They Would Give to Others- II

Themes/Subthemes	Number of Participants Who Reported Theme	
	Currently Pregnant ($n = 3$)	Post-Pregnancy ($n = 21$)
Information about the Postpartum Period	0 (0%)	2 (10%)
Hire a postpartum doula for help right after birth	0	1
Seek medication adjustment early for PPD	0	1
Ensure that you get enough sleep	0	1
Additional Reflections	0 (0%)	4 (19%)
I wish I had found more hopeful/positive information about BD and pregnancy	0	3
Was not diagnosed with BD prior to pregnancy	0	1

Coping with challenging aspects of pregnancy or considering becoming pregnant. Table 8a and 8b present the two themes representing the aspects of pregnancy that participants found most challenging or believed to be most challenging when considering pregnancy. The coping strategies they used or believe would be effective in helping them to manage these challenges is presented as well.

Most challenging aspects of being pregnant or considering becoming pregnant. Of the entire sample, 42 percent indicated that the most challenging aspect of having BD and being pregnant or considering becoming pregnant was managing their own worries. Participants reported worrying about a variety of issues, including the teratogenic effects of medication, experiencing a mood episode, and the genetic risk of their children developing BD.

Ways that participants coped or would cope with the most challenging aspects of being pregnant or in considering becoming pregnant. Of the entire sample, 26% of participants indicated that they coped with the most challenging aspects of having BD and being pregnant or considering becoming pregnant by using self-care strategies to manage stress. Participants reported using a variety of stress reduction strategies, including positive thinking (such as using positive self-talk and reminding oneself that things will be okay), being more aware of moods, journaling, praying, and getting adequate sleep. For example, one participant (#2) reported the following:

> Getting up every 2 hours to pee and then trying to get comfortable *again* is difficult for anyone. Doing it for months at a time *really* messes with your sleep cycle, and not long after, your mood. I try to allow myself a longer period of time to sleep—usually 12 hours, so that I get closer to the 7-8 hours I *need*. Also, *no naps* . . . I may need a nap every couple of weeks but I only take short (30 minute) power naps and only early in my day. Some days I am so tired I sit on the couch most of the day. But at least I am not up all night by myself while the rest of the world sleeps.

Nine participants said that having a strong support network helped them cope or could help them to cope with the challenges of BD and pregnancy. One participant (#36) commented, "As much as my family tries to understand, they don't really know; they can't 100% relate. That's why joining a bipolar support group or bipolar pregnant or a mother group could be comforting." Another participant (#38) reported that at times she has felt too depressed to leave her home and attend appointments with her psychiatrist; however, if necessary, her psychiatrist will make medication adjustments after having her clients telephone or text message their symptoms to her. This participant found her psychiatrist to be very supportive and effective.

One participant (#32) stated that she worried she would decide to become pregnant due to poor judgment and recklessness during a hypomanic episode. She stated that she copes with this by using an intrauterine device and having an agreement with her husband that they will discuss pregnancy with her psychiatrist before they attempt to become pregnant.

Table 8a

Most Challenging Aspects of BD and Pregnancy

Subthemes	Number of Participants who Reported Theme		
	Pre-Pregnancy ($n = 14$)	Currently Pregnant ($n = 3$)	Post-Pregnancy ($n = 21$)
Worrying (about teratogenic effects of medication, experiencing a mood episode, genetic risks to child)	8	1	7
Controlling mood episodes	1	1	5
Switching/foregoing medication/taking different medication	4	0	3
Deciding whether or not to have children	4	0	1
Lacking information about BD and pregnancy	2	0	1
Lacking social support	0	0	2
Dealing with stigma from self and others	2	0	
Not being diagnosed with BD prior to pregnancy	0	0	2
N/A, did not experience any challenges	1	0	1
Receiving incorrect advice from healthcare providers lacking expertise in BD	0	0	1
Pregnancy hormones	0	0	1
Inability to sleep through the night	0	1	0

Table 8b

What Helps One Cope Effectively With the Challenges of BD And Pregnancy

Subthemes	Number of Participants who Reported Theme		
	Pre-Pregnancy ($n = 14$)	Currently Pregnant ($n = 3$)	Post-Pregnancy ($n = 21$)
Using stress reduction techniques (positive thinking, prayer, journaling, getting adequate sleep)	5	2	3
Having a strong social support system (including joining a support group and talking with people)	2	0	7
Talking with my doctor or psychiatrist	2	0	3
Taking medication	0	0	3
Participating in psychotherapy	1	1	1
Learning about BD including how to parent a child with BD	2	0	1
Using an IUD to prevent unplanned pregnancy	0	0	1
Becoming pregnant at a more age-appropriate time	0	0	1
Adopting or using a surrogate	1	0	0
Nothing can help	0	0	1

Stress reduction and complementary medicine methods participants tried or would consider trying to help manage BD during pregnancy. Table 9 presents the coping and complementary medicine methods participants used or would consider using in order to help to manage their BD during pregnancy and the postpartum period and the coping methods participants used or would considering using to help manage their mood during pregnancy. The most common methods were psychotherapy, massage, and meditation or mindfulness ($n = 11$, 10, and 9, respectively).

about postpartum psychosis as well as postpartum depression. She also expressed her

wish that healthcare providers would screen for postpartum mania and family history of

BD, in addition to screening for postpartum depression. One participant (#38) reported

that she had taken St. John's wort to treat her depression and it caused her to become

manic; she believed it was important that the safety of herbal medicine be discussed in an

informational resource on BD and pregnancy. Another participant (#37) shared her

strategy for communicating with her psychiatrist: She reported that she would keep a note

card in her wallet and write down her medication questions whenever she thought of

them. She would then discuss these questions at her next appointment. It helped her to

remember her concerns and use her time more effectively.

Table 10

Other Information Women Would Like Included in an Informational Resource about BD and Pregnancy

Subthemes	Number of Participants who Reported Theme		
	Pre-Pregnancy (*n* = 14)	Currently Pregnant (*n* = 3)	Post-Pregnancy (*n* = 21)
Medication teratogenic effect rates compared to environmental risks so that the risks are easier to deduce	1	0	0
Infertility and BD	1	0	0
How to create a plan with one's partner regarding symptoms of	1	0	0
BD and how to manage them	0	0	0
Post-delivery psychiatric care information	0	0	1
Parenting books and recommendations	0	0	2
ECT information	0	0	2
Positive information about BD and pregnancy	0	0	2
Directory of OBs with psychiatric expertise	0	0	1
Early signs of BD in children	1	0	1
The pros and cons of herbal medicine	0	0	2

Chapter V

Discussion

Introduction

The purpose of this study was to explore the questions and concerns of women with BD regarding pregnancy with BD. Whereas there is much information available to the public regarding the general treatment of BD, little information is available on the comprehensive and holistic management of BD during pregnancy. Clinical psychology can provide unique perspectives and behavioral strategies, which can create a more complete, usable, and helpful body of knowledge. This study hoped to fill a gap in the literature with an aim to making the body of knowledge regarding mental health interventions and existing research into an informational resource, such as a self-help workbook, that would be accessible to nonprofessionals.

This section will reflect on the key findings of my study with respect to the existing literature on BD and pregnancy and on professional collaboration in BD, as well as implications and limitations. Regarding validity, participants appeared to be interested, engaged, and honest when disclosing their opinions and concerns. In particular, although no financial or other incentive was provided to participants, they remained on the telephone with me for an hour or more, and they provided lengthy and thoughtful responses to the fill-in questions in the survey. Participants reported that they found the topic of pregnancy issues related to BD to be an area of considerable importance to them and that they wished to share their concerns with me. Several participants reported that they hoped to help other women with BD avoid the frustration they themselves had experienced.

Key Findings

Several key findings emerged from my study. They include the fact that (a) women diagnosed with BD are profoundly concerned about pregnancy issues, (b) women with BD are afraid of harming their children, (c) women with BD are eager to educate themselves about pregnancy issues, and (d) they are dissatisfied with the information they are finding. In addition, (e) women with BD want their healthcare providers to inform them of the risks associated with various treatment options during pregnancy, as well as pregnancy and mood issues; (f) women with BD recommend and desire psychotherapy during pregnancy, and they want to know how to include their partners in therapy; and (g) women with BD are concerned about their relationships with their healthcare providers. Details about these findings are provided in this section.

Women diagnosed with BD are profoundly concerned about pregnancy issues. The majority of participants reported experiencing significant anxiety regarding the various aspects of BD and being pregnant or considering becoming pregnant, and they reported that they spent a great deal of time worrying about these issues. Participants expressed a variety of concerns, including the risks becoming pregnant might pose to their mood and mental stability, the uncertainty associated with teratogenic effects of psychotropic medications, and whether or not to stop taking medication or change their medication regimens. Given the fact that it is common for women who are *not* diagnosed with BD or other significant illnesses to demonstrate a great deal of anxiety regarding pregnancy issues, it is not surprising that women with BD would be even more anxious and have greater concerns than usual about pregnancy. This finding supports the results of Paterson et al. (2013), in which women with BD demonstrated more concerns about the effects of pregnancy on their moods than did women with unipolar depression. A few of the participants in my study seemed unaware that their BD symptoms could be affected by pregnancy and vice versa; this finding was particularly surprising and concerning, as it has been recommended that all women diagnosed with BD during or prior to their reproductive years be educated about pertinent issues related to pregnancy and BD (Barnes & Mitchell, 2005).

Women with BD are afraid of harming their children. Many participants expressed fears that the associated issues related to their condition of BD might cause them to hurt their unborn children or the children they had previously given birth to. Women reported the fear that taking medication during pregnancy or breastfeeding while under medication could cause short- or long-term damage to their babies. They were also afraid that they might harm their unborn children due to mood episodes. They worried that they might become suicidal or homicidal during depressive or manic episodes and kill themselves, their babies, or their older children.

Participants in this study also reported being concerned that their parenting skills might be negatively affected by future mood episodes. This finding was supported by the research of Paterson and colleagues (2013) who also found that it was common for women with BD to be worried about parenting, and that as a group they reported being motivated to be more vigilant parents because of their BD. Many of the participants reported experiencing great trepidation and deep-seated guilt over the ethicality of taking the risk that they might pass BD on to their children given the genetic heritability of the disorder. Trippitelli et al. (1998) found that the majority of couples with a partner with BD that were considering pregnancy would take advantage of genetic testing if it were available in order to obtain early intervention for their children to help reduce the risk of their experiencing mood episodes. Meiser et al. (2007) found that women with BD often held fears about passing BD on to their children and that there were significant associations between these fears, perceived stigma of BD, and their being less willing to have children.

Women with BD are eager to educate themselves about pregnancy issues, and they are dissatisfied with the information they are finding. Almost all participants reported that they actively sought information about the ways in which BD could affect pregnancy, as well as how to best prepare for and manage these risks during the various stages of pregnancy. They wanted to know how to best increase the likelihood that their own health as well as the health of their babies would be maintained. Participants reported that they would first ask their healthcare providers for answers to their questions about BD and pregnancy. If they were not able to obtain the answers they were looking for, they would often use the Internet as a source for the desired information. They would search for credible, medically supported information. Many women reported that they found it very difficult to find information they could trust and that was geared toward women with BD rather than towards healthcare professionals. When women could not find what they were looking for on websites that were written by professionals or health care establishments, they would often then resort to using peer-support websites. They would also look to other women with BD who had previously been pregnant for advice and information about their experiences. This finding has been reflected in postings to Facebook support groups, such as Bipolar, Depressed, and Pregnant or a Mother (2013), in which pregnant women ask each other for advice about changing their medication regimens, for example. It is important to note that participants who had never

been pregnant and who were not sure if they wanted to have children also actively sought

information about pregnancy. Women in the precontemplative stage of pregnancy likely

have less access to obstetricians and might want to gain a basic understanding of BD and

pregnancy issues before addressing the topic with their psychiatrists and physicians.

Women with BD want their healthcare providers to explain the risks

associated with various treatment options during pregnancy to them, as well as

pregnancy and mood issues. Most participants expressed the desire to learn about the

most up-to-date findings on any teratogenic effects of medications used to manage mood.

Several participants also described interest in complementary medicine, such as herbal

treatments for mood. A few participants wanted to learn about other medical options,

such as ECT and TMS. They also wanted to know about the relative risks of

experiencing mood episodes during pregnancy and the postpartum period. Several

women wondered how they could best prepare themselves for pregnancy, as well as

wanting information regarding post-delivery psychiatric care. Many participants voiced

concerns and questions about how changing hormone levels associated with pregnancy

and the postpartum period might affect-mood and symptoms of BD. The lack of

availability of such important information reported by these women is a finding

supported by Studd and Nappi (2012), who suggested that even psychiatrists are often

fairly uninformed about these issues. They stated that many psychiatrists never screen

for reproductive causes of depression, and they also stated that it was much more

common for psychiatrists to prescribe antidepressants rather than hormonal treatments.

Women with BD recommend and desire psychotherapy during pregnancy,

and they want to know how to include their partners in therapy. Many participants who participated in individual psychotherapy or counseling during pregnancy and the postpartum period reported that they found it helpful to them and they recommended that other pregnant women with BD do the same. Several of the participants who had never previously given birth stated that they would most likely want to participate in psychotherapy should they become pregnant. Many participants also reported that they would find it comforting to be able to speak with other women with BD who had previously been pregnant; they expressed a desire to engage with others in support groups for pregnant women and mothers with BD. Psychotherapy could be beneficial to pregnant women with BD, as it could help them to cope with the stress and anxiety associated with pregnancy, improve their ability to effectively interact with their treatment team, regulate their mood by keeping their sleep cycles consistent, and monitor new mood symptoms that might occur. This finding is supported by a large body of evidence which indicates that many different forms of psychotherapy may help to improve the course of BD, including overall functioning, relationship functioning, and overall life satisfaction (Miklowitz et al., 2007). A few participants said they believed their partners could also benefit from support groups or couples counseling, so that they could learn how to best support participants during pregnancy. They wanted to know how to include their partners in therapy.

Women with BD are concerned about their relationships with their healthcare providers. Several participants emphasized the need to establish a team of trusted healthcare providers who collaborate with each other well during their pregnancy. They reported that it was important to have one's therapist and medical providers networked with each other because physicians and psychiatrists tended to be less accessible to clients. They emphasized the importance of finding providers with expertise, knowledge, and experience with BD and pregnancy issues. Several participants reported experiencing stigma and misinformation from their healthcare providers regarding pregnancy issues; for example, some participants were told that women with BD should not conceive.

A few participants reported a perception that healthcare providers considered them to be undesirable patients due to the risks associated with their pregnancies. The finding that certain healthcare providers may hold stigmatized views of people with BD is supported by Smith and Cashwell (2010), who found that it was very common for healthcare professionals who lacked mental health training, education, and experience to hold more negative attitudes toward people with mental illness. They also found that healthcare professionals who were undergoing clinical supervision tended to hold less stigmatizing attitudes toward people with mental illness.

Implications of Findings

Implications for psychological interventions, medical interventions, and policy based on the findings of this study are discussed in this section.

Implications for psychological interventions. Many women who participated in this study stated that they experienced a great deal of anxiety regarding pregnancy issues. Psychotherapy could help women with BD to address their anxiety, learn coping skills to deal with stress, monitor themselves for emergent BD symptoms, and better manage their moods.

Group psychotherapy. Several participants alluded to a sense of isolation regarding the experience of having BD and being pregnant or considering becoming

pregnant. In-person and online support groups that facilitate connections between

pregnant women and new mothers with BD could be particularly helpful to them. They

may feel more understood by other women going through the same difficult experience.

Perhaps more mental health clinicians should work to create and run these support groups.

Participant recruitment efforts might focus on advertising via flyers and pamphlets in

obstetricians' waiting rooms and at pregnancy classes. There is existing research and

evidence that group therapy can be an effective way to improve the course of BD (Castle

et al., 2010). Four of the 10 mothers with BD interviewed by Venkataraman and

Ackerson (2008) expressed a desire for more support groups for mothers with BD so that

they could get advice about parenting from others dealing with the unique challenges

associated with having a BD diagnosis.

Couples psychotherapy. Many participants expressed concerns that new mood

symptoms associated with pregnancy could strain their relationships with their partners.

Indeed, existing literature indicates that people with BD are very likely to end up

divorced, and one study found that 18% of marriages ended following postpartum

episodes of psychosis (Blackmore et al., 2013; Walid & Zaytseva, 2011). Couples

therapy could be particularly helpful to pregnant women with BD and their partners, as it

could improve communication between the couple, address and repair marital problems,

and help the partner to be more supportive to the woman with BD who is pregnant.

Family psychotherapy and parenting interventions. Many of the participants in

this study expressed concerns about the way that BD might affect their parenting skills.

Participants wondered if there were steps they could take to minimize the chance that their offspring developed BD. They also wanted to learn about the early signs of BD so that they could obtain treatment for their children early on if necessary. There is some evidence that it may be possible to identify prodromal symptoms of BD in children (Hauser & Correll, 2013). Preliminary research has also demonstrated that children of parents with BD have more severe behavioral problems than average and that interventions designed for parents with BD may improve their children's observed behavior problems (Jones et al., 2013). Parents with depressive and hypomanic episodes have been found to be at a greater risk of having children who develop BD (Miklowitz, et al., 2013). There is evidence that family-focused therapy, in which children and their family members are taught to recognize early symptoms of mood episodes and intervene with them, as well as improve family members' communication and problem-solving skills, may improve mood symptoms in children at high risk for developing BD later in life. Thus, family psychotherapy and parenting interventions could address the fears of women with BD by improving their parenting skills and offering support regarding the possibility that their children may develop BD.

Implications for medical interventions. First and foremost among the implications of this study for medical practitioners is the need for healthcare providers to educate their patients with BD about typical pregnancy concerns. Table 11 lists typical concerns that women with BD may have regarding pregnancy based on this study's findings. Healthcare providers should consider addressing these issues with their patients; otherwise, findings from this study suggest that women with BD are likely to search for answers on their own, from both official and peer support websites, which may not necessarily provide accurate information.

Table 11

Patient Education Checklist for Healthcare Providers

Teratogenic effects of medications used to treat BD during pregnancy and nursing

Risk of mood episodes during pregnancy and the postpartum period

The effects of changing hormone levels associated with pregnancy on mood

Genetic risks of children developing BD

The effects of BD on parenting skills

How to decide whether or not to have children

How to educate and involve one's partner in being supportive regarding BD and pregnancy

Referrals to psychotherapists and/or online and in-person support groups

Psychosocial methods to improve one's mood stability during pregnancy

Links to informational websites to learn more about BD and pregnancy

---

In addition, there appears to be a great need for multidisciplinary collaboration, especially between psychologists and physicians, when treating patients with BD who are pregnant. Given the high anxiety that women with BD face regarding pregnancy issues, it may be useful for healthcare providers to refer these patients to psychologists, social workers, and other mental health clinicians who can provide psychotherapy and take the time to help these women express and better cope with their anxieties and fears. Ideally, the therapist, psychiatrist, and obstetrician would consult regularly and openly as a team in order to share key concerns and thus more effectively address the individual woman's specific needs. Fleury et al. (2012) found that comprehensive services and continuity of care were key factors in the recovery of people with mental illness; these factors were associated with a decreased number of emergency room visits and hospitalizations.

Some strategies that were found to improve multidisciplinary collaboration included establishing stronger informal networks between practitioners of diverse backgrounds, having a strong commitment to patient empowerment, and the development of electronic medical records.

Moreover, there appears to be a need for medical education programs to teach trainees about stigma toward patients with mental illness. Results from this study highlighted the fact that some women with BD feel that their healthcare providers hold stigmatized views of people with mental illness. Some reported that their providers gave them the impression that women with BD should not have children. These results are consistent with past research. For example, one prior study demonstrated that nearly half of the women with BD who engaged in genetic counseling were advised against pregnancy. This is much higher than the rate at which experts on BD would advise against pregnancy (Viguera, 2005). The fact that women with BD often feel that those who they approach for help are either ill informed or hold biases towards their illness is not a healthy situation for them or their unborn children. Perhaps schools that educate medical personnel, including medical schools and nursing schools, should make it a priority to provide training on stigma as it relates to mental illness. Practitioners should become more aware of their biases toward people with mental illnesses, including women with BD who wish to conceive. They should be aware of the ethical dilemmas posed by the risk of passing BD on to one's descendants and educated about the capacities of women with BD to be good parents with sufficient support (Groisman, Mathieu, & Godard, 2012). It also may be beneficial for healthcare practitioners to be more sensitive to the way that they present information about pregnancy to women with BD; several participants reported that they had the impression that the information available about BD and pregnancy was solely focused on risks and worst-case scenarios, and this increased their anxiety even more.

Another implication of these findings concerns physicians who treat women with BD. These practitioners may want to consider referring women with BD to psychiatrists with perinatal expertise to help manage their mood and medication during pregnancy. Several participants in this study recommended that other women with BD look for healthcare practitioners with experience treating BD during pregnancy. Given the complexity of the decisions that must be made, associated uncertainties, ever changing information available, and the overall high-risk nature of helping women with BD manage pregnancy, it is logical that the more training, knowledge, expertise, and experience a healthcare provider has in this area, the better the chances will be of them effectively helping their patients. Those with expertise in perinatal psychiatry, a specialty area of psychiatry that focuses on pregnancy issues among women with mental illnesses, have expressed concerns that many psychiatric residency programs do not adequately prepare future psychiatrists to treat pregnancy issues competently (Freeman, 2009). Therefore, general practitioners and family physicians should strongly consider referring their pregnant patients with BD to psychiatrists, preferably those with perinatal experience and training.

Implications for policy. It would be beneficial to offer contraception counseling to women with BD who are in their reproductive years, as it could reduce their chance of having unplanned pregnancies, which can pose a variety of risks to the health of the mother and child. It may be particularly important to provide support and education to women with BD who do not wish to become pregnant and who experience unprotected sex associated with mania, so that they can develop plans to decrease their risk of unwanted pregnancy.

Recent research findings indicate that postpartum psychosis is most common on the day of delivery; therefore, it may be beneficial for women diagnosed with BD to remain at the hospital until at least 1 day after giving birth (Harlow et al., 2007). This would allow women to be monitored and screened for symptoms of psychosis by medical professionals during the period of highest risk. If such an event is caught in time, treatment could be implemented immediately, preventing potentially catastrophic effects on the mother or infant.

Private and public health insurance organizations should be aware of the high-risk nature of pregnancy for women with BD. More psychotherapy and psychiatric resources should be made available to women with BD who are pregnant or who have given birth in the past year. Government-funded childcare discount programs should be made available to women with BD who face financial hardship. The postpartum period has been found to be the highest mood episode risk period in a woman's lifetime, and it is therefore important to find ways to help these women protect their sleep and minimize stress (Curtis, 2005).

Limitations

Given the exploratory nature of this study, an open-ended question format was utilized to allow participants to provide the widest array of possible responses. The respondent burden associated with this question format may have accounted for the online survey's high dropout rate, and it is possible that the high dropout rate could have limited the generalizability of the findings. For example, the participants who remained in the study until the end may have been more concerned about issues related to BD and pregnancy, more articulate and comfortable expressing their ideas online, and had more free time than the average woman with BD. A larger participant sample may have revealed more information.

In addition, participants' diagnoses were not confirmed with structured clinical measures; however, it was believed that attempting to administer these measures could have discouraged participation, as such an interview would have greatly increased the time demand and no incentive was provided to participate. Participants were recruited via the Internet, either through Craigslist or Facebook. Therefore, the results obtained may not be representative of all women with BD. The participant sample could be more computer savvy, younger, and perhaps have a higher socioeconomic status (SES) than the average woman with BD. Craigslist advertisements were posted in major cities, which could have created a more metropolitan sample, which may have more access to psychiatric resources. These recruitment methods could have prevented women with BD of lower SES, lower education level, and more advanced age from accessing the survey and providing their perspectives on the issues addressed.

Future Research

Overall, this study revealed that women with BD are very concerned about pregnancy issues, and they are afraid of how factors associated with BD may harm their children. The contributions from this study can hopefully inform healthcare providers about the types of information women with BD seek, thereby improving treatment outcomes for this high-risk population. It is heartening to learn that quite a bit of research on the topic of BD and pregnancy as well as postpartum depression has been

conducted in the past few years. Hopefully this trend will continue. An informational

resource aimed toward women with BD, which contains the information these

participants found crucial, would be useful in helping them to develop a more realistic

understanding of the various issues they need to consider in making the important

decision about whether or not to have children and how to ensure the safety of

themselves and their children should they decide to have them.

Printed in the USA
CPSIA information can be obtained
at www.ICGtesting.com
LVHW011634311223
767720LV00085B/3196